Immunology
AN OUTLINE FOR STUDENTS OF MEDICINE AND BIOLOGY

Immunology

AN OUTLINE FOR STUDENTS OF MEDICINE AND BIOLOGY

D. M. Weir, M.D., M.R.C.P. (EDIN.)

Immunology Laboratory, Department of Bacteriology
University of Edinburgh Medical School

FOURTH EDITION

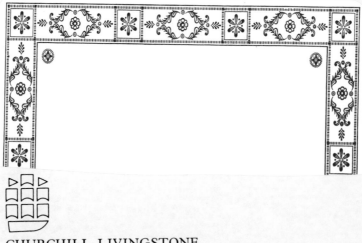

CHURCHILL LIVINGSTONE
EDINBURGH LONDON AND NEW YORK 1977

CHURCHILL LIVINGSTONE
Medical Division of Longman Group Limited

Distributed in the United States of America by
Longman Inc., 19 West 44th Street, New York, N.Y.
10036 and by associated companies, branches and
representatives throughout the world.

First Edition   1970
Second Edition   1971
  Reprinted   1972
Third Edition   1973
Fourth Edition   1977

ISBN 0 443 01522 8

First–3rd editions published under title:
Immunology for Undergraduates

British Library Cataloguing in Publication Data
Weir, Donald Mackay
    Immunology.—4th ed.
    I. Immunology
    I. Title II. Immunology for undergraduates
    616.07'9   QR181   77–30004

Printed in Singapore
Singapore Offset Printing (Pte) Ltd

Preface to the Fourth Edition

This new edition previously appeared under the title *Immunology for Undergraduates* and the present revision is the fourth edition of the text. *Immunology for Undergraduates* over the last seven years had proved of value to a wide range of students and graduates in biology and medicine, and this new edition has been extensively revised and rearranged to cover the needs of such readers. Much new material has been introduced, including discussion of genetic influences in the immune response, and there is a new section on laboratory tests used in clinical immunology. All the figures have been redrawn and a number of new ones included. The aim of this volume is to provide an outline of the subject without extensive description of experimental background and unnecessary detail. Many exceedingly complex situations have been highly simplified, and the hope is that accuracy has not been sacrificed for clarity.

In the author's view the reader new to immunology should be provided with a simplified, comprehensible picture of the subject based upon a clear understanding of the basic principles which will provide an outline structure for the thoughtful reader to build upon and, in the light of subsequent knowledge, perhaps even to come to different conclusions.

Thanks are due to the many colleagues who have made constructive suggestions for improvements in the text and to Miss Daphne Lytton for redrawing the figures with skill and imagination. The index was prepared by Dr Valerie Inglis. I wish to thank Dr Caroline Blackwell for editorial assistance.

1977 D. M. Weir

Contents

1

Immunity

THE SCOPE OF IMMUNOLOGY

The tissues and cells capable of exhibiting what is now recognized as an adaptive immune response have an evolutionary history of some 400 million years and the forms taken by the response during this period have maintained a remarkable constancy both at the molecular and at the functional level. The basic pattern of the protein molecules involved has been retained, with the diversification that has occurred through evolutionary selective pressures being superimposed on this basic pattern.

Recognition

Immune phenomena as expressed in the higher animals have evolved from **recognition mechanisms** that enabled a multicellular primitive animal to distinguish between itself and other foreign species – this idea of **self-non-self discrimination** lies at the foundation of immunological theory. Self-recognition mechanisms appear very early in evolution and can be seen in marine organisms, such as sponges. Reaggregation of dispersed colonies is regulated by species specific surface glycoproteins. Failure of adhesion of unrelated species amounts to a primitive form of graft rejection. The cells lining the cavity of sponges are able to capture microorganisms present in the water drawn into the cavity, and phagocytosis (p. 12) plays a role in the metamorphosis of insects in removing dead and disintegrated tissue.

An important recognition phenomenon occurs in the interaction between pollen grains and plant stigma, which appears to depend on the nature of surface proteins. Pollination and germination only occur if the pollen and stigma are genetically compatible and self-fertilization is prevented.

Primitive marine species such as sea stars and corals appear to be able to reject grafts of unrelated forms. Self-non-self discrimination enables the maintenance of **specific partnerships** between cells of a multicellular organism and provides an organism with the additional benefits of recognizing and excluding changed self-constituents and potentially harmful parasitic organisms, such as fungi and bacteria. The particular cell surface molecules that are recognized and determine foreignness are often carbohydrates or glycoproteins. The recognition factors themselves are proteins and it is interesting to note that the production of one of the recognition proteins (immunoglobulin M, p. 52) of the higher vertebrates is specifically stimulated by carbohydrate molecules. Immunoglobulin M is believed to represent the precursor of all the other forms of **immunoglobulin** and has its origin in the most primitive vertebrate fishes.

This has led to the view that there is a continuity between the primitive ability to recognize carbohydrates of foreign cell surfaces and the highly developed recognition factors found in higher vertebrates, which are able to discriminate between a variety of organic molecules of carbohydrate and non-carbohydrate nature.

Immunity

The meaning of the term 'immunity' as it is used today derives from its earlier usage referring to exemption from military service or paying taxes. It has long been recognized that those who recovered from epidemic diseases such as smallpox and plague were exempt from further attacks and such immune individuals were often used in an epidemic to nurse those suffering from active disease. In England the procedure of cow-pox vaccination developed by Edward Jenner in 1798 for protection against smallpox and that used by Francis Home in Edinburgh for measles protection were essentially empirically measures performed without understanding of the underlying principles.

The foundations for an understanding of immunity were laid by the invention of the microscope, the recognition of microorganisms and the advent of Pasteur's **germ theory of disease**. Pasteur's chance observation that aged cultures of chicken cholera bacillus would not cause the expected disease in chickens led to the development of methods for reducing the virulence of pathogenic microorganisms called **attenuation**. The protection given to animals by preinoculation of such attenuated organisms led to the widespread use of the method for immunization purposes.

The discovery of the tubercle bacillus by Robert Koch led him to describe the phenomenon of delayed hypersensitivity or **cell-mediated immunity** as it is known today. Immunology as a science began with the demonstration by von Behring and Kitasato at the

Koch Institute in Berlin in 1890 of an antibacterial substance or factor in the blood of animals immunized against tetanus and diphtheria organisms. The neutralizing ability of such blood serum for the bacterial toxins was the first demonstration of the effect of what is now recognized as antibody globulin.

The part played by **phagocytic cells** in clearing away and destroying bacteria was recognized by Metchnikoff, a Russian biologist working in France. Later the helpful effect of antibody (called opsonins by Almroth Wright) in encouraging phagocytosis became apparent thus reconciling two opposing schools of thought on immune mechanisms – one believing the process to be brought about completely by blood factors and the other upholding an entirely cellular viewpoint.

Pfeiffer and Bordet demonstrated the activity of a serum factor called **complement**, which, participates with antibody in the destruction of bacteria and has now been shown to have a wide variety of important biological activities. Paul Ehrlich proposed the first theory of antibody formation – **the side chain theory.** This proposed the existence of receptors on the surface of cells that could be released into the blood and neutralize bacterial toxins.

Antibody specificity

The specificity of antibody for the agent (i.e. the antigen) which induced its formation led to the use of antibody as an analytic tool. Thus the antigenic characters of bacterial and non-bacterial substances could be worked out and systems of classification of microorganisms were developed on this basis. Landsteiner used antibody-antigen interaction to define the **ABO blood group system** on the basis of antigenic differences in red cell membranes, and was also responsible for performing the ground work on the chemical basis of antigenic specificity.

Self and non-self

In more recent years with increasing knowledge of the molecular processes underlying the functioning of cells it became possible to formulate theories on the mechanisms whereby the tissues and cells responsible for producing antibody performed this function. The need for such theories became apparent with the recognition of human diseases where the immune mechanisms had become deranged and were treating the individual's own tissues as if they were foreign antigens. Thus the question of how the immune system distinguished between what was foreign and what was part of self became important and resulted in the formulation of new theories to explain these phenomena, notable among which was the **clonal selection** theory of Burnet. These attempted to define the scope and limitation of Ehrlich's 'contrivances by means of which the immunity reaction ... is prevented from acting against the organism's own elements and so giving rise to autotoxin'. The advances made in this area gave a new dimension to the science of immunology which until then was devoted almost exclusively to the prevention of.infectious disease by vaccination and immunization. This new field of study – **immunobiology** – has drawn the attention of biologists to the apparent central importance of immune mechanisms in the evolution of multicellular animals.

The cells of the immune system are probably derived from the primitive cellular defence mechanism that arose with the evolution of the invertebrates. This is manifested by the engulfment and walling off of foreign particles. The phagocytic cells responsible for this do not respond by proliferation so that the animal does not become better adapted to deal more effectively with the foreign material (p. 37). It is doubtful if the immune response, as it is recognized today, first appeared with the need for protection from parasitic microorganisms but evolved in the primitive vertebrates as a way of protecting themselves from their parasitic relatives. In the absence of such protection the parasite could attach itself to a host and because the tissues of the two animals were so similar the host would be unable to react against the parasite which would thus be accepted rather like a piece of successfully grafted compatible tissue (chap. 7). Burnet who is one of the main exponents of this view has suggested that the mechanism that underlies the protective response to parasites depended on the host making its own tissues antigenically different from the parasite so that the parasite could be recognized as foreign. The evolution of a defence mechanism able to resist parasitic invasion would have the added advantage of treating in the same way any tissues of the animal that changed their cell surface antigens. This, as will be discussed later (chap. 11), is a characteristic of many tumour cells and the employment of the immunological defence mechanisms to rid the body of such cells would confer a clear evolutionary advantage to the species.

Immunity and genetics

Knowledge of the genetic control of protein synthesis is likely to make considerable advances as a result of the study of the synthesis of immunoglobulins. The concept that **two genes** may code for a **single polypeptide chain** and that groups of closely linked genes may be basic units of mammalian genomes have emerged from studies on immunoglobulin synthesis.

It is now recognized that interaction between different cell types may exert control over protein synthesis affecting for example the particular class of immunoglobulin being manufactured by a lymphocyte (chap. 4). The study of immunoglobulin structure has shown that in the human there are at least 10 different types and that each type contains an enormous number of variants differing slightly from each other in amino acid sequence.

The gene complex of the mouse that controls the cell surface antigens important in transplantation (graft) rejection has proved to be an invaluable general model for the study of the **major**

Table 1.1 Development of immunology, vaccination to the present day

	Immunity	
Late eighteenth century	Smallpox vaccination – Jenner	
Late nineteenth century	Germ theory of disease, attenuated and killed vaccines – Pasteur Tubercle bacillus and cell-mediated immunity – Koch Antitoxins against diphtheria and tetanus – von Behring, Kitasato Complement activity – Pfeiffer, Bordet Agglutination of bacteria – Durham Side chain theory of immunity–Ehrlich Phagocytosis and cellular immunity – Metchnikoff	

	Immunochemistry	Immunobiology
	Blood groups – Landsteiner Antigenic determinants – Landsteiner, Heidelberger, Marrack	Antiglobulin test – Coombs, Mourant, Race Recognition of autoimmunity
Mid-twentieth century	Electrophoretic separation of gamma globulin – Kabat, Tiselius	Clonal selection theory of immunity – Burnet (Jerne)
	Structural analysis of antibody molecule – Porter, Edelman	Immunological tolerance – Medawar, Owen (Glenny) Transplantation immunology, Tumour immunology, Rhesus immunization, Deficiency states, role of the thymus
Present day	Relationship between structure and biological activities of immuno-globulin molecule and genetic control mechanisms Determinants of immuno-genicity of antigen molecule	Immunogenetics and evolution of immune system Lymphocyte activation and products, cell cooperation Role of macrophages – antibacterial, and cytotoxic effects

transplantation antigen systems of higher vertebrates. More recently the small segment of chromosome 17 that contains this gene complex has evoked considerable interest among geneticists and immunologists. They have recognized that in addition to controlling cell surface antigens, there are closely linked genes that determine differences in level of antibody responses to many antigens, differences in susceptibility to tumour viruses and a number of other important immunological traits (chap. 9). This gene complex is now the most thoroughly and extensively characterized segment of chromosome in any mammalian species and as such it constitutes a very valuable model for studies of gene evolution, gene action and organization.

Technical advances

Modern biochemical techniques have helped to add precision and sensitivity to immunological methods. These include the use of radioisotopes to measure accurately the primary binding of antibody with antigen and to demonstrate the metabolic activity of cells engaged in antibody production. Protein fractionation techniques and peptide analysis of the antibody molecule have thrown light on the chemical basis of specificity of the molecule and the relationship of structure to function as well as confirming a genetic basis for antibody formation and providing factual limitations on earlier theories of antibody formation.

The understanding of immunological processes underlying the reaction of the body to tumours, to transplanted tissues and organs and to infectious agents has gained much ground as the result of these advances in immunochemical techniques. Clinical developments have included the recognition of **autoimmune** and **immunological deficiency** diseases and the feasibility of **organ transplantation**. Technical advances in the study of the *in vitro* behaviour of cells of the immune system and in the quantitation of serum proteins have provided valuable diagnostic help in the recognition and management of these clinical situations. Phylogenetic studies have stimulated investigations into the development and control of the lymphoid tissues leading, for example, to a new understanding of the role of that previously enigmatic organ, the thymus.

Thus it can be seen that immunity in its original meaning, referring to resistance to invasion by a parasite by means of a specific immune response, is only one activity of a cellular system in animals. The total activity of the cellular system is concerned with mechanisms for preserving the integrity of the individual with far-reaching implications in embryology, genetics, cell biology, tumour biology and many non-infective disease processes.

The subject of immunology can be considered under three general headings: **immunity**, dealing with the adaptive response to infective agents; **immunochemistry**, concerned with the chemical nature of antigens and antibodies; and **immunobiology**, which encompasses a variety of topics of biological importance and deals with the activity of the cells of the immune system and their relationship to each other and their environment.

FURTHER READING

Brock, T. (Ed.) (1961) *Milestones in Microbiology*. Part III, Immunology, pp. 121–144. Englewood Cliffs, N.J.: Prentice-Hall.

Burnet, F. M. (1969) *Changing Patterns*. New York: Elsevier.

Foster, W. D. (1970) *A History of Medical Bacteriology and Immunology*. London: Heinemann.

Good, R. A. (1976) Runestones in immunology: inscriptions to journeys of discovery and analysis. *J. Immunol.*, **117**, 1413.

Herbert, W. J. & Wilkinson, P. C. (1977) *A Dictionary of Immunology*. Oxford: Blackwell.

McNeill, W. H. (1976) *Plagues and Peoples*. Oxford: Basil Blackwell.

Parish, H. J. (1965) *A History of Immunization*. Edinburgh: Livingstone.

2

Innate immunity: non-specific defence mechanisms

The healthy individual is able to protect himself from potentially harmful microorganisms in the environment by a number of very effective mechanisms present from birth which do not depend upon having previous experience of any particular microorganism. The innate immune mechanisms are **non-specific** in the sense that they are effective against a wide range of potentially infective agents. The main determinants of innate immunity seem genetically controlled, varying widely with species and strain and to a lesser extent between individuals. Age, sex and hormone balance play lesser roles. In comparison, acquired immune mechanisms, discussed below, depend upon the development of an immune response to individual microorganisms that is specific only for the inducing organism.

Determinants of innate immunity

Species and strain
Marked differences exist in the susceptibility of different species to infective agents. The rat is strikingly insusceptible to diphtheria whilst the guinea-pig and man are highly susceptible. The rabbit is particularly susceptible to myxomatosis and man to syphilis, leprosy and meningococcal meningitis. Susceptibility to an infection does not always imply a lack of resistance because although man is highly susceptible to the common cold he overcomes the infection within a few days. Dogs in contrast are not susceptible to the virus agents responsible for the common cold in man. In some diseases, although a species may be difficult to infect (i.e. insusceptible), once established the disease can progress rapidly (i.e. lack of resistance). For example rabies, although common to both man and dogs, is not readily established as the virus does not easily penetrate healthy skin. Once infected, however, the resistance mechanisms in both species are not able to overcome the disease. Marked variations in resistance to infection between different strains of mice have been noted.

Table 2.1 Determinants of innate immunity

Specific host determinants	Physical determinants	Active anti-microbial determinants
Species and strain	Skin and mucous membrane barriers, moist surfaces	Antibacterial and antifungal secretions of skin – sweat and sebaceous secretions
Individual genetic factors	Anatomical traps, e.g. nasal cavity	
Age		Antibacterial and anti-viral secretions of mucous membranes
	Mechanical cleansing, e.g. cilia	
		Antimicrobial substances of tissue fluids, e.g. lysozyme, basic polypeptides
Hormonal balance		Phagocytosis and digestion

In man the habits and environment of a community affect its ability to resist particular infections by acquired immune mechanisms developing early in life. This environmentally determined type of resistance is easily confused with the genetically controlled innate immunity and makes it difficult to establish differences in innate immunity in different communities. It is, however, fairly clear that the American Indian and the Negro are more susceptible to tuberculosis than are Caucasians. It seems reasonable to assume that certain interspecies and interstrain differences have arisen by a process of natural selection.

Individual differences and influence of age
The role of heredity in determining resistance to infection is well illustrated by studies on tuberculosis infection in twins. If one homozygous twin develops tuberculosis, the other twin has a three to one chance of developing the disease compared to a one in three chance if the twins are heterozygous. Sometimes genetically controlled abnormalities are an advantage to the individual in resisting infection as for example in a hereditary abnormality of the red blood cells (sickling) which are less readily parasitized by *Plasmodium falciparum* thus conferring insusceptibility to malaria. Infectious diseases are more severe at the extremes of life, and in the young animal this appears to be associated with immaturity of the immunological mechanisms affecting the ability of the lymphoid system to deal with and react to foreign antigens. In the elderly, on

the other hand, physical abnormalities (e.g. prostatic enlargement leading to stasis of urine) are a common cause of increased susceptibility to infection.

Nutritional factors and hormonal influences
The adverse effect of poor nutrition on susceptibility to infectious agents is usually not seriously questioned. Experimental evidence in animals has shown repeatedly that inadequate diet may be correlated with increased susceptibility to a variety of bacterial diseases and this has been associated with decreased phagocytic activity and leucopenia. In the case of infective agents such as viruses, which depend upon the normal metabolic function of the host cells, malnutrition, if it interfered with such activities, would be expected to hinder proliferation of the potentially infective agent. There is experimental evidence in support of this view in a number of animal species, which when undernourished were less susceptible to a variety of viruses including vaccinia virus and certain neurotropic viruses. The same may be true of malaria infections in man. The parasite requires para-amino benzoic acid for multiplication and this may be deficient when a low level of nutrition exists. The exact role of nutritional factors in resistance to infectious agents in man is difficult to determine by epidemiological data. Poor diet is often associated with poor environmental conditions and increased incidence of infection can correlate with poor sanitary conditions.

There is increased resistance to infection in diseases such as diabetes mellitus, hypothyroidism and adrenal dysfunction. The reasons for this have yet to be elucidated in detail, but it is known that the glucocorticoids are anti-inflammatory agents, decreasing the ability of phagocytes to digest ingested material (probably by stabilizing the lysozomal membranes).

Mechanisms of innate immunity

Mechanical barriers and surface secretions
The intact skin and mucous membranes of the body afford effective protection against non-pathogenic organisms and a high degree of protection against pathogens (Fig. 2.1). The skin is the more resistant barrier because of its outer horny layer. The damp surface of the mucous membranes of the respiratory tract acts as a trapping mechanism and, together with the action of the hair-like processes or cilia, sweep away foreign particulate material so that it passes into the saliva and then is swallowed. On reaching the stomach the acid gastric juices destroy any microorganisms present. Nasal secretions

SKIN

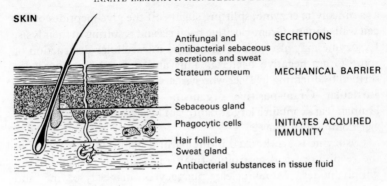

Antifungal and antibacterial sebaceous secretions and sweat	SECRETIONS
Strateum corneum	MECHANICAL BARRIER
Sebaceous gland	
Phagocytic cells	INITIATES ACQUIRED IMMUNITY
Hair follicle	
Sweat gland	
Antibacterial substances in tissue fluid	

RESPIRATORY MUCOUS MEMBRANE

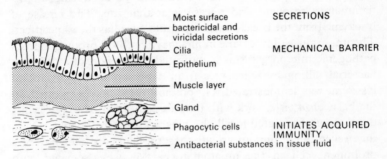

Moist surface bactericidal and viricidal secretions	SECRETIONS
Cilia	MECHANICAL BARRIER
Epithelium	
Muscle layer	
Gland	
Phagocytic cells	INITIATES ACQUIRED IMMUNITY
Antibacterial substances in tissue fluid	

Fig. 2.1 Innate immune mechanisms.

and saliva contain mucopolysaccharides capable of inactivating some viruses and the tears contain lysozyme active against Gram-positive bacteria. The sebaceous secretions and sweat of the skin contain bactericidal and fungicidal fatty acids and these constitute a very effective protective mechanism against potentially pathogenic microorganisms. Certain areas of the body such as the soles of the feet are deficient in sebaceous glands and this explains in part why such areas are susceptible to fungal infection. The protective ability of these secretions varies at different stages of life and it is known that fungal 'ringworm' infection of children disappears at puberty.

Bactericidal substances of the tissues and body fluids
Lysozyme. This is a low molecular weight basic protein found in relatively high concentration in polymorphonuclear leucocytes as well in most tissue fluids except CSF, sweat and urine. It functions

as a mucolytic enzyme, splitting sugars off the glycopeptides of the cell wall of many Gram-positive bacteria and resulting in their lysis. Lysozyme may also play a role in the intracellular destruction of some Gram-negative bacteria. This antibacterial agent was described by Fleming in 1922 who was able to measure its effect on a particular Gram-positive organism, *Micrococcus lysodeikticus*. Human tears contain a large quantity of lysozyme and egg white is a rich commercial source.

Lysozyme is synthesized in the parotid gland, in the mucosa of the respiratory and gastrointestinal tracts and in the spleen and lymph nodes. Mononuclear phagocytes make lysozyme and polymorphoniclear granulocytes contain lysozyme but do not synthesize it. Thus protection by lysozyme is brought about by its local synthesis and release into the mucous secretions and by mononuclear phagocytes that infiltrate a tissue during an inflammatory response and release it at that site. The release of lysozyme from the breakdown of granulocytes has the same effect. The importance of lysozyme in phagocytic cells in protection from pathogenic microorganisms is indicated by a report of a defect in bacterial killing by leucocytes from a person in whom lack of lysozyme was demonstrated. The possibility has been suggested, on the basis of *in vitro* work with tumour cells exposed to lysozyme, that lysozyme secreted locally by macrophages may play a role in the prevention of tumour growth. Macrophages are known to be a prominent cell in the inflammatory response associated with tumours.

Basic polypeptides. A variety of basic proteins, derived from the tissue and blood cells damaged in the course of infection and inflammation, have been found in the tissues of animals. This group includes spermine and spermidine, which kill tubercle bacilli and some staphylococci, and the arginine and lysine containing basic proteins protamine and histone. The ability of these basic polypeptides to destroy bacteria probably depends on the ability of the NH_2 groups to react non-specifically with the nearest acidic substance.

Phagocytosis and the inflammatory response

Microorganisms or inert particles such as colloidal carbon entering the tissue fluids or blood stream are very rapidly engulfed by various circulating and tissue-fixed phagocytic cells. These cells are of two types, the **polymorphonuclear** leucocytes of the blood – or microphages as they are sometimes called – and the **mononuclear** phagocytic cells distributed throughout the body both **circulating** in the blood and **fixed** in the tissues. The latter cells make up the cells of the reticuloendothelial system or RES and are given the generic name macrophages. Macrophages in the blood are known as monocytes, those in the connective tissues as histiocytes, those in the spleen, lymph nodes and thymus as the sinus-lining macrophages (sometimes called reticulum cells). It is now established that the macrophages of connective tissues are derived from the peripheral blood monocytes as are the Kupffer cells of the liver, the alveolar macrophages of the lungs, and the free macrophages of the spleen, lymph nodes and bone marrow. In the spleen and lymph nodes, both free and fixed macrophages occur in close association with the reticular cells, which act as a framework for the macrophages. The reticular cells themselves, although able to ingest particulate material, are not regarded as mononuclear phagocytes, nor are the dendritic cells (p. 34) of the follicles of the spleen and lymph nodes. The term **mononuclear phagocyte system** to describe actively phagocytic cells is now widely accepted as a more satisfactory description of the function, origin and morphology of phagocytes than the older RES classification, which included actively and poorly phagocytic cells.

The three essential features of these phagocytic cells are (1) that they are actively **phagocytic**, (2) that they contain **digestive enzymes** to degrade ingested material and (3) that the macrophages are an important **link** between the innate and the acquired immune mechanisms, partly by passing on antigens or their products to the lymphoid cells and partly by retaining antigens to ensure that lymphoid cells are not overwhelmed by excess antigen (p. 64).

The process of phagocytosis is undoubtedly one of the earliest accomplishments of living cells. At the beginning of the century Metchnikoff in Russia first appreciated the continuity of this function through evolution and the important role of this activity in resistance to infectious agents.

The role of the phagocyte in innate immunity is to engulf particulate (phagocytosis) or soluble material (pinocytosis) and either to digest it or if indigestible to store it away so that it no longer serves as a local irritant, e.g. carbon particles from a polluted atmosphere.

The macrophages of the mononuclear phagocyte system serve a very important role in clearing the blood stream of foreign particulate material such as bacteria. The efficiency of this process can be dramatically illustrated by injecting colloidal carbon into the circulation of a mouse. Samples of blood taken at short intervals thereafter show a very rapid removal of most of the particles within a few minutes after injection and the blood is completely cleared by 15 to 20 minutes. Dissection of the animal will show massive localization of the carbon particles, particularly in Kupffer cells of the liver, of the spleen sinus-lining macrophages and in the macrophages of the lungs. This system of phagocytic cells has an enormous capacity to take up material from the blood and the finding of free microorganisms in the blood stream usually means that there is a continued release of organisms from an abscess or from the bacterial 'vegetation' found in bacterial endocarditis.

There are many examples of the ability of the phagocytic cells of animals to ingest and dispose of different kinds of microorganisms. The destruction of phagocytic cells by chemical agents in the rabbit results in the animal losing resistance to a normally avirulent pneumococcus. The enhanced ability of macrophages from animals infected with tubercle bacilli or listeria to resist these and other infective agents is discussed on page 123. Some microorganisms such as brucellae and streptococci can resist intracellular digestion (p. 118).

The way in which phagocytes **recognize, bind** and **ingest** particulate materials such as microorganisms is only beginning to be understood. Initial adherence depends on two distinct mechanisms. (1) Relatively non-specific binding that appears to depend, as shown by work in the author's laboratory, on cell surface glycoproteins of the phagocyte binding to cell wall carbohydrates of the microorganism. This ability is probably derived from the recognition abilities found in primitive species discussed in Chapter 1 and has been retained during evolution. (2) More recently evolved mechanisms that utilize receptors in the phagocyte cell membrane for a part of the antibody molecule (Fc component, p. 51) and for a component of the complement system (C3b, p. 17). Microorganisms coated with antibody and complement thus adhere to the phagocyte and can then be ingested. Antibodies can markedly enhance the activities of phagocytic cells and even improve intracellular digestion. Such antibodies are known as **opsonins** (p. 56). Injury to tissue excites an inflammatory response consisting of dilation of local capillaries, slowing of the blood flow and exudation of oedema fluid, and phagocytic cells which initially stick to capillary walls then pass through the walls of these more permeable vessels. Once outside the capillaries the phagocytic cells, which are initially mainly the polymorphonuclear leucocytes of the blood, migrate to the source of the irritation. This leucocyte attraction phenomenon is known as **chemotaxis** and can readily be induced by microorganisms entering the tissues, by the breakdown products of damaged tissue cells and by various irritant substances (possibly acting in this way because they bring about damage to cells). The precise mechanisms of chemotaxis are not understood but it is known that complexes of antigen and antibody generate the production of a diffusible factor which also acts in this way; this phenomenon requires the participation of complement components (p. 19).

After the initial polymorph infiltration in an inflammatory response, the mononuclear cells (blood macrophages) can be seen to enter the area but very little is known at present about the nature of the mechanisms which lead to the accumulation of these cells. The process seems to be quite distinct from that responsible for polymorph migration (see p. 73).

Once ingested, susceptible bacteria disintegrate within an hour or two partly because of the secretion of acids and digestive enzymes secreted into the vacuole surrounding them. The cytoplasmic granules (lyosomes) of polymorphs contain many enzymes including acid and alkaline phosphatase, β glucuronidase and ribonuclease. The antibacterial agents lysozyme (p. 11) and phagocytin are also present. These cytoplasmic granules fuse with the vacuole containing the microorganism.

Phagocytin. Extracts of the cytoplasm of polymorphonuclear leucocytes from several species have been found to contain an acid soluble protein bactericidal to Gram-negative bacteria and also to a few Gram-positive organisms. Phagocytin is present together with other antibacterial substances in the granules of polymorphs.

Temperature

The temperature dependence of many microorganisms is well known and tubercle bacilli, pathogenic for mammalian species, will not infect cold-blooded animals. Hens which are naturally immune to anthrax can be infected if their temperature is lowered. Gonococci are readily killed at temperatures over 40°C and fever therapy was a common treatment of gonococcal infection before the introduction of antibiotics.

It is therefore apparent that temperature is an important factor in determining the innate immunity of an animal to some infective agents and it seems likely that the **pyrexia** which follows so many different types of infection can function as a **protective** response against the infecting microorganisms. Recent evidence shows that human lymphocytes cultured at 39° and 41°C show enhanced responsiveness to plant haemagglutinins (p. 73) and streptococcal products.

The complement system

The existence of a heat labile serum component with the ability to lyse red blood cells and destroy Gram-negative bacteria has been known for the last 50 years or so. The chemical complexity of the phenomenon was not initially appreciated by early workers who ascribed the activity to a single component – **complement**. It is now known that complement is in fact an extremely complex group of serum proteins present in low concentration in normal serum. Collectively the complement system is the effector mechanism responsible for the biological activity of complement-fixing antibodies (p. 54).

Complement components have the characteristic of interacting with certain antibody molecules once these have combined with antigen. These components are best known for their ability to combine with anti erythrocyte antibody attached to the red cell membrane, the effect of complement being to bring about lysis of the red cell by what appears to be enzymic digestion of small areas of the cell membrane. Much of what is known today about the complement system comes from studies of immune haemolysis.

Complement, together with the blood clotting, fibrinolytic and kinin generating systems, are triggered enzyme cascade systems. The first three complement components, Cl, 4 and 3, circulate in an inactive form as proenzymes and are converted to their active form by their predecessors in the cascade. Complement components are not all synthesized by a single type of cell and are all fairly large proteins, C3 being the most abundant with a concentration of about $1200 \mu g/ml$ serum. The intestinal epithelium, macrophage, liver and spleen are the main sources of the components.

An outstanding feature of the activation of the **classical complement pathway** is the fragmentation or cleaving of individual components into **large** fragments, which enter into combination with other complement components, and **small** fragments, which have other biological activities described later.

There are three separate stages involved in the activation of the complement system with **C3 activation** as the central event. It is usual in the complement literature to show a bar over the complement enzymes and activated components formed during the activation process, e.g. C567, but this has been avoided here for simplicity.

1. The **recognition stage** involves an interaction between the first component of complement C1 (the recognition unit) and a complement binding site on an immunoglobulin molecule.. The complement binding site is not available on the native Ig molecule and becomes exposed after conformational changes in the molecule following interaction with antigen. The complement binding site is present in the Fc fragment of the immunoglobulin molecule (see p. 54) and in the IgM molecule has been found to be associated with a particular part of the Fc fragment called the CH_3 domain (p. 51).

   The C1 component is made up of three distinct proteins held together by calcium ions C1q, C1r and C1s. C1q is the recognition protein and binds to the exposed site on the Fc fragment of the immunoglobulin molecule. It is believed that C1q binding induces conformational changes in the C1 complex resulting in conversion of C1r to an enzyme capable of activating C1s.

2. The **activation stage** in which activated C1s acts on C2 and C4 components resulting in the production of a C2, C4 complex known as C3 convertase. This enzyme then acts on C3 and splits C3 into a small and a large subunit, C3a and C3b. C3a is released into the body fluids. C3b in association with its activating enzyme forms another enzyme, C5 convertase, and this leads on to the last stage.

3. The **membrane attack** stage. This occurs when the recognition and activation stages have taken place on the surface of a cell such as an erthrocyte, used in *in vitro* serological tests with complement, or on a bacterium invading the tissues. This membrane attack sequence is initiated by the reaction of C5 convertase on the next complement component C5. Once again a small fragment C5a is split off and released into the body fluids. A larger C5b fragment remains bound to the activating complex. This leads to the incorporation of the remaining complement components C6-9 without further enzymic action and consequent lysis of the red cell or bacterium. The biochemical events associated with the interaction of these later components with the C1425 complex are not understood but are thought to be due to an effect on a phospholipid component of the cell membrane. The result is the production of nearly circular holes 80-100A in diameter in the red cell membrane and loss of its contents (Fig. 2.2).

Recently a new pathway for the activation of complement components has been described. This **alternate** or **by-pass**

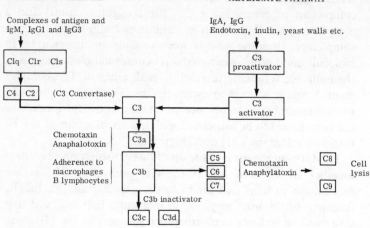

Fig. 2.2 Simplified view of activation of complement pathways and activities of components.

pathway misses out the C1, C4 and C2 components and starts at the C3 step. The components C3–C9 are depleted when this pathway is activated although for some unknown reason the system is poorly lytic. This alternate pathway is independent of the Fc portion and can be initiated by aggregated immunoglobulin (IgG, IgA and possibly IgE) or $F(ab)_2$ fragments (see p. 50) and also by various polysaccharides including endotoxin, zymosan and agar. These substances, in the presence of magnesium ions, convert C3 proactivator into C3 activator, which splits C3 into the small C3a subunit and the large C3b subunit.

Uncontrolled activation of the complement system is avoided in part by the lability of the activated components and by several serum proteins that limit activation. These include a C1 esterase inhibitor and the important controlling protein C3b inactivator that cleaves C3b into at least two fragments, as shown in Figure 2.2.

Red cell lysis whilst the most intensively studied complement activity is by no means the only role played by the complex. Complement action is of some considerable importance because of its ability to neutralize various types of cell such as human cells or Gram-negative bacteria after they have interacted with antibody. Complement appears to render the bacteria susceptible to lysozyme. Tumour cells for example can survive indefinitely in the presence of antibody but on the addition of complement the cells develop blebs in the membrane, become fragile and lose many of their intracellular constituents leading to death of the cell. Another extremely important role of complement is in the attraction of polymorphonuclear phagocytes to sites of antigen-antibody interaction. This important step in the inflammatory process is known as **chemotaxis** and appears to depend on the components C5, 6 and 7 interacting with the C1,4,2,3 complex. C3a and C5a also have a chemotactic effect. In hypersensitivity states (chap. 6) complement activation is responsible for the formation of substances known as **anaphylatoxins**, three of which are identifiable by MW differences (7,500, 8,500 and 10,000). They arise after C3 and C5 activation and are responsible for bringing about the release of histamine leading to increased vascular permeability and smooth muscle contraction. The formation of the plasma kinins, e.g. C-kinin, which are active in hypersensitivity states, also appears to depend upon complement activation. Complement components C1–C3 are concerned in promoting phagocytosis and act as **opsonins** (p. 56). Table 2.2 shows some of the biological effects of activation products of the complement system.

Many cells of the lymphoid system have receptors for complement components. Macrophages and B lymphocytes (p. 591), for example, react with split products of C3 (C3b), which may play a

Table 2.2 Biological effects of activation products of complement system

Complexes and components involved	Activities
C1, 4	Neutralization of herpes simplex virus together with IgM
C1, 4, 2	Possible generation of kinins, increase in vascular permeability
C3b	Leucocyte phagocytosis Immune adherence, C3b on rbc, wbc or platelet adheres to normal rbcs – agglutination (*in vitro*) Viruses coated with Ig and complement adhere to platelets or rbcs resulting in removal by phagocytes
C3a	Leucocyte chemotaxis Anaphylatoxin (contraction of smooth muscle, increased vascular permeability and histamine release)
C5a	Leucocyte chemotaxis Anaphylotoxin
C5, 6, 7	Leucocyte chemotaxis
C8, 9	Cytotoxic effect

part in triggering the activation of the lymphocyte and in phagocytosis by macrophages of antigen-antibody complexes with bound complement.

Normal human serum as noted above contains an inhibitor (an α_2-neuraminoglycoprotein) of C1 esterase. This inhibitor may be quantitatively or qualitatively deficient and lead to the condition known as hereditary angioneurotic oedema. The effects are probably due to the formation of anaphylatoxins with the consequent release of histamine. Complement deficiencies are rare, but hereditary deficiencies of the C1 components, C2 and C4 are accompanied in many cases by a variety of chronic diseases, including recurrent infections and renal disease. In laboratory practice complement lysis tests have wide and important applications (p. 182).

FURTHER READING

Austen, K. F. (1974) The immunobiology of complement. *Transpl. Proc.*, **6**, 1.

Bacteriological Reviews (1960) Symposium on mechanisms of non-specific resistance to infection. *Bacteriological Reviews*, **24**, 1.

van Furth, R. (1975) *Mononuclear Phagocytes in Immunity*. Oxford: Blackwell.

Howard, J. G. (1963) Natural immunity. In *Modern Trends in Immunology I*, ed. by Cruickshank, R. London: Butterworth.

Mackaness, G. B. & Blanden, R. V. (1967) Cellular immunity. *Progr. Allergy*, **11**, 89.

Müller-Eberhard, H. J. (1975) Complement. *Ann. Rev. Biochem.*, **44**, 697.

Nelson, D. S. (1976) *Immunobiology of the Macrophage*. New York: Academic Press.

Schur, P. H. & Austen, K. F. (1968) Complement in human disease. *Ann. Rev. Med.*, **19**, 1.

Vogt, W. (1974) Activation, activities and pharmacologically active products of complement. *Pharmacol. Rev.*, **28**, 125.

3

Antigens

Antigens are substances of various chemical types capable of stimulating the immune system of an animal to produce a response specifically directed at the inducing substance and not other unrelated substances. The specificity of the immune response for chemical structures (antigenic determinants) of the antigen molecule is an important characteristic. An antibody directed against an antigenic determinant of a particular molecule will react only with this determinant or another **very similar** structure. Even minor chemical changes in the determinant with the resulting change in shape will markedly alter the ability of the determinant to react with antibody. The term antigen, referring to substances capable of acting as specific stimulants of the immune response or reacting with antibody in an *in vitro* serological test, is used rather loosely by immunologists.

Immunogens and haptens
Substances which *de novo* are capable themselves of inducing an immune response are sometimes referred to as **immunogens** and are usually large molecules. In contrast, substances (often simple chemicals) incapable alone of inducing an immune response are termed **haptens**. To induce an immune response the hapten requires to be attached to a carrier molecule (usually a serum protein such as albumin). The hapten molecule then acts as a determinant of antigenic specificity and is referred to as an **antigenic determinant**. Immunogens also have antigenic determinants which are simply particular chemical groupings within the macromolecule.

Specificity and cross reactions
It is important at this point to distinguish clearly between structural specificity of an antigenic determinant and its distribution specificity. For example the ubiquitous nature of the glucose molecule – present in many different types of macromolecule –

21

must be distinguished from its specific chemical structure. An immune response against a glucose determinant in antigen AG would be likely to react also with glucose in antigen BG provided the two determinants are equally accessible. The antibody directed against the glucose determinant is not as is sometimes thought a non-specific type of antibody but is simply reacting with an identical chemical determinant in another antigen molecule. A typical cross reaction is with pneumococcal polysaccharide type S–V111 which has a tetrasaccharide repeating unit containing cellobiuronic acid alternating with an isomer of lactose. Antisera to such a structure will cross react with oxidized cotton cellulose containing cellobiuronic acid residues.

Heterophile and Forssman antigens

In laboratory serological practice, **cross reactions** are a common source of difficulty, and cross reactivity is often found between antisera to certain bacterial antigens and antigens present in cells such as erythrocytes. Antigens shared in this way are known as **heterophile antigens** and antisera to these will cross react with cells or fluids of many different species of animal and with various microorganisms. The chemical determinants responsible for this cross reactivity are not known but are presumed to be similar or identical groupings possibly of mucopolysaccharide and lipid nature present in large structural molecules. The best known of the heterophile antigens is the **Forssman** antigen which is present in the red cells of many species as well as in bacteria such as pneumococci and salmonellae. Another heterophile antigen is found in *E. coli* and human red cells of group B. Another important example is the cross reaction between *Treponema pallidum* and an extract of mammalian heart–**cardiolipin**. The common shared antigenic structures are phosphatidylglycerols differing only in their fatty acid side groups. Cardiolipin, being more readily available than *Treponema pallidum*, serves as a useful antigen in the serological tests for syphilis (p. 191).

Carbohydrate, lipids, nucleic acids and protein antigens

It is common to classify antigens as protein polysaccharides or lipids; this is, however, an oversimplified view as although many molecules of entirely protein, polysaccharide or lipid nature are antigens it is also not infrequent to find carbohydrate moieties as determinants on protein or lipid macromolecules or peptide units as determinants on polysaccharide macromolecules.

Carbohydrate determinants are commonly found in the cell wall of bacteria, and antibodies to these determinants are used for grouping the organisms. Streptococcal cell walls contain such antigens, and group A organisms have N-acetylglucosamine as the predominant determinant. In contrast group C streptococci have N-acetylgalactosamine as the main determinant. Pneumococci also contain polysaccharide in their capsules and the biological importance of these is discussed in Chapter 8.

Lipids and nuclei acids in purified form are not good at inducing an immune response and have to be complexed with a larger molecule or altered in some way before they do so. For example, nucleic acids conjugated to methylated bovine serum albumin can induce antibody formation. Nucleic acids as antigens are of some interest to immunologists as anti nucleic acid antibodies are found in patients with the disease systemic lupus erythematosus (see p. 147).

Proteins are highly complex molecules and have featured prominently in immunological studies because of their wide distribution in nature and their ready availability in highly purified form. Unfortunately in the present state of knowledge of the antigenic determinants of protein molecules so little information is available about the precise nature of the peptides acting as determinants in different protein macromolecules that immunologists still describe antigens in terms of the whole molecule, e.g. bovine serum albumin (BSA) rather than the individual determinants of specificity within the macromolecule.

Antigenic determinants
Degradation, chemical modification and synthesis of determinants
The number of determinants (sometimes referred to as its valency) in a molecule like BSA is probably in excess of 18 although only about six of these are exposed in the native intact molecule. The other (hidden) determinants can be identified only when the molecule is broken down by, for example, enzyme hydrolysis. Antibody produced in response to injection of the whole molecule appears to be able to react with the fragments produced by hydrolysis, and it therefore appears that the molecule is broken down into similar fragments after injection. This might be brought about by the digestive enzymes in phagocytic cells (p. 13).

Attempts to identify the chemical nature of antigenic determinants have used this type of degradation procedure with some degree of success and some insight has been gained into the size and other features of the determinants. Two other approaches have also been used – chemical modification of known determinants and synthesis of polyamino acid and polysaccharide antigens.

Degradation studies have been carried out on silk fibroin, a linear polypeptide chain of molecular weight between 50,000 and 60,000. The determinant site capable of reacting with antibody appears to consist of between eight to 12 amino acids (27–44Å) with the C terminal tyrosine making a considerable contribution to the site. The important role of **tyrosine** is further supported by the finding that the poor antigen gelatin can be made antigenic by the addition of tyrosine in which the native molecule is very deficient. The possibility that tyrosine confers rigidity on the gelatin molecule has been suggested (see also p. 27).

The protein coat of tobacco mosiac virus consists of identical subunits (approx. 2000) each with a molecular weight of about 16,500 consisting of 158 amino acids. The antigenic determinant site is present in the chain between position 108 and 112 and, unlike fibroin, contains no aromatic amino acids. The hydrophobic nature of leucine appears to be an important characteristic of this particular determinant site.

The blood group substances are large molecules consisting of about 75 per cent polysaccharide and 25 per cent polypeptide. Degradation studies have shown that the substances owe their specificity to groups at the end of the carbohydrate chains, for example, A substance specificity is determined by α-N-acetylgalactosaminoyl – (1–3) – galactose.

Foreignness

A substance which acts as an antigen in one species of animal may not do so in another because it is represented in the tissues or fluids of the second species. This underlines the requirement that an antigen must be a **foreign** substance to elicit an immune response. For example, it follows that egg albumin whilst an excellent antigen in the rabbit, fails to induce an antibody response in a fowl. The more foreign a substance is to a particular species the more likely it is to be a powerful antigen. A good antigen need not contain different building blocks, e.g. amino acids of a protein, but their arrangement should be such that at least part of the surface of the molecule presents a configuration which is unfamiliar to the animal. Since macromolecules have a three dimensional structure, it is easy to visualize how they could become unfolded by denaturation so as to present new and unique surface arrangements.

Foreignness can be a property which depends on chemical groupings which are entirely unfamiliar to the animal. Arsonic acid, for example, can be introduced by diazotization into a protein molecule. Such a group is known as a **hapten** and acts as the **determinant** of the **antigenic specificity** of the molecule, the protein to which the hapten is attached functioning simply as a **carrier molecule.**

Karl Landsteiner in the early part of this century carried out very extensive studies on the antigenic specificity of such hapten chemical determinants resulting in a new appreciation of how critical and precise was the fit between antibody and an antigenic determinant. Landsteiner's work with, for example, the arsonic acid determinant (AsO_3H_2) showed that changes, even as minor as the replacement in the benzine ring, of the AsO_3H_2 group by a

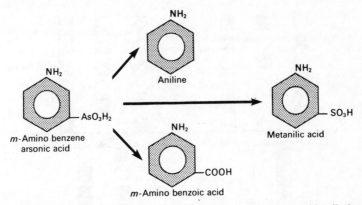

Fig. 3.1 Rabbit antisera to azoproteins containing any of the above acid radicals as antigenic determinants react only with the inducing azoprotein and not with any of the others. Even azoproteins obtained by changing the $-COOH$ of *m*-amino benzoic acid or the $-SO_3H$ of metanilic acid to the ortho or para positions do not react with antisera to the original determinant. Methyl and halogen radicals substituted in the benzene ring instead of the acid radicals shown in the figure are less effective as determinants of specificity and considerable cross reactions are found in precipitin tests.

COOH or a SO_3H group (Fig. 3.1) was sufficient to affect substantially the ability of azo proteins containing the determinant, to react with antibody against the unchanged hapten.

The influence of changes in shape brought about without the removal or substitution of groups is shown by studies with stereoisomers of macromolecules containing tartaric acid where the antibody to L tartaric acid fails to combine with its isomer D tartaric acid. It was concluded from studies of this type (a) that **acidic** and **basic** groups are very important in regulating the specificity of an antigenic determinant, (b) that **spatial** configuation of haptens is important, (c) that **terminal** groups in an antigen are often important determinants of specificity and (d) that **interchange** of non-ionic groups of similar size had little effect on specificity of a determinant.

It became clear from studies of this type that a very slight variation in the chemical constitution or even shape of a molecule could substantially affect the ability of antibody to combine with it. Despite this knowledge immunologists even today are still far from understanding the chemical nature of the determinant groups in complex proteins and polysaccharides. Studies by Sela in Israel with synthetic polypeptides show that the **surface arrangements** of the amino acids in a branched polyamino acid structure are critical as determinants of antigenic specificity (Fig. 3.2).

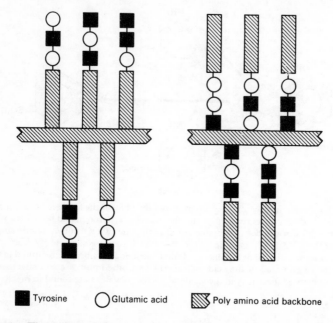

■ Tyrosine   ◯ Glutamic acid   ▨ Poly amino acid backbone

Fig. 3.2 The amino acids, tyrosine, glutamic acid can convert a non-antigenic polyamino acid branched structure (polyalanine and polylysine) into an antigen provided they are attached to the outer end of the branches (left); if attached at the inner end of the branches (right) the complex is not antigenic.

If the three dimensional structure of a protein is altered by heating or other form of denaturation, it is no longer able to combine as effectively with antibody to the original native molecule. Enzymes act as antigens and RNAse molecules after oxidation become unfolded and the change in shape prevents the interaction of the molecule with antibody to native RNAse.

Immunogenicity

Molecular size

For a substance to be antigenic in its own right (i.e. an immunogen) without the need to be attached to a carrier molecule, requires that it has certain properties which have not yet been fully defined. Amongst these is the fact that **high molecular weight** materials are better antigens than those of low molecular weight but above a certain threshold it does not appear to be a determining factor. A substance below a molecular weight of about 5000 is not likely to be a good antigen. This phenomenon may be partly explained by the presence in a larger molecule of repeating antigenic determinant groups, and in a complex molecule of a large variety of potential determinants, one or more being capable of preferentially stimulating an immune response. Large molecular size alone is not sufficient to confer antigenicity on a substance. Synthetic polymers of many types can be built up into large macromolecules and are non-antigenic. The polyamino acid backbone (polyalanine and polylysine) of the molecule shown in Figure 3.2 is non-antigenic and only becomes capable of inducing an immune response by the addition of further different amino acids. It has been suggested that the lack of antigenicity of synthetic polymers is due to their lack of internal molecular complexity. Thus the antigenicity of naturally occurring macromolecules may be due to their many different low molecular weight constituents giving complexity to the molecule. Tyrosine has been found to be a helpful constituent for a polypeptide to be a good immunogen although this amino acid is not essential. In general, aromatic amino acids consistently enhance the immunogenicity of a polypeptide.

Physical state, shape, change

Some low molecular weight chemical substances appear to contradict the need noted above that an antigen be a large molecule. Among these are included picryl chloride, formaldehyde and drugs such as aspirin, penicillin and sulphonamides. These substances are highly antigenic, particularly if applied to the skin. The reason for this appears to be that such materials form **complexes** by means of covalent bonds with tissue protein, and the complex of these substances, acting as haptens with tissue protein carrier, forms complete antigen. This has important implications in the development of certain types of hypersensitivity states (p. 105).

The physical state of a protein antigen can affect its antigenicity. The same substance, e.g. the serum protein BSA, in aggregated and aggregate-free form can show wide divergence in ability to stimulate immunity, the aggregated form being strongly antigenic in the rabbit while the aggregate-free form induces a specific state of unresponsiveness (immunological tolerance, p. 64). This knowledge of the influence of **particle size** has been applied to production of antisera to snake venoms. The venom (neurotoxin) of low molecular weight and thus poor immunogenicity was linked to carboxymethylcellulose resin. The toxin-resin complex was non-toxic and highly immunogenic in rabbits.

Some molecules carry what is sometimes called 'built-in-adjuvanticity', which means that they have the capacity to stimulate the cells of the antibody system in a non-specific manner so that they are able to handle antigen more effectively. Bacterial endotoxin produces this effect as also do *Bordetella pertussis* organisms, and these materials can enhance the antigenicity of a weak antigen if administered at the same time. The effect seem likely to be due to a powerful 'triggering' effect by bacterial endotoxin on a particular lymphocyte population (B cells, see p. 60) responsible for making antibody. In human immunization the efficacy of the 'triple vaccine', diphtheria, pertussis, tetanus, is partly due to the effect of *B. pertussis* (p. 137).

Polysaccharide antigen, for example dextran of molecular weight (MW) 600,000, is a good antigen, whereas a dextran of MW 100,000 is not. There is no obvious reason for this as the two materials are made up of identical building blocks and do not differ as far as the type of antigenic determinant is concerned.

The effect of electric charge of a molecule on its immunogenicity has been studied and found to be unrelated to its ability to induce an immune response. Polypeptides in which the net charge was zero elicited comparable amounts of antibody as charged polypeptides.

The shape of a polypeptide molecule does not affect its ability to elicit an antibody response and linear polypeptides which have no organized conformational structure can be potent immunogens.

Persistence of antigen

The ability of an animal to **degrade** a polysaccharide antigen can affect its immune reactivity to the antigen. Some pneumococcal polysaccharides appear to be resistant to digestion in the mouse and in sufficient dose are able to mop up antibody as it is made, resulting in the absence of detectable antibody in the serum. The same effect can be produced if the antigen is protected in some way from the tissue fluids and inflammatory cells. This can occur if the material is incorporated in oil as an emulsion (see p. 43) or is walled off by fibrous tissue. The antigen dose, form, route of entry and host determinants are discussed in Chapter 4.

FURTHER READING

Barrett, J. T. (1974) *Textbook of Immunology*. 2nd edition. London: Kimpton.

Borek, F. (1972) Molecular size ans shape of Antigens. In *Immunogenicity*, p. 45, ed. Borek, F. Amsterdam: North Holland.

Boyd, W. C. (1963) *Fundamentals of Immunology*. London: Inter-science.

Dumonde, D. C. (1965) Tissue specific antigens. *Adv. Immun.*, 5, 30.

Gill, T. J. (1972) The chemistry of antigens and its influence on immunogenicity. In *Immunogenicity*, p. 5, ed. Borek, F. Amsterdam: North Holland.

Heidelberger, M. (1956) *Lectures in Immunochemistry*. New York: Academic Press.

Kabat, E. A. (1968) *Structural Concepts in Immunology and Immunochemistry*. New York: Holt, Rinehart & Winston.

Landsteiner, K. (1945) *The Specificity of Serological Reactions*. Cambridge, Mass: Harvard University Press.

Sela, M. (1965) Immunological studies with synthetic polypeptides. *Adv. Immun.*, 5, 30.

Sela, M. (Ed.) (1975) *The Antigens*. New York: Academic Press.

4

Acquired immunity

Microorganisms which overcome or circumvent the innate non-specific immune mechanisms come up against the host's second line of defence. To give expression to this form of immunity it is necessary that antigens of the invading microorganisms come in contact with cells of the immune system (macrophages and lymphocytes) which leads to the initiation of an **adaptive immune response** specific for the inducing antigen. This response takes two forms, which usually develop in parallel and, although discussed separately, are closely related as both depend upon cells of the lymphoid system.

1. **Humoral immunity.** The characteristic of this form of immunity is the appearance in the blood of globulins known as antibodies or immunoglobulins. These combine **specifically** with the antigen which stimulates their production and can lead to some remarkable consequences. For example, the antigen molecules or particles may be clumped, their toxicity may be neutralized, their uptake and subsequent digestion by phagocytes facilitated and cellular antigens that are part of a cell surface such as a red blood cell or bacterium may be lysed.

2. **Cell-mediated immunity.** Lymphoid cells may be induced by prior exposure to antigen, to react subsequently directly with the inducing antigen and bring about **cytotoxic** effects, as for example on foreign cells from a graft. The precise manner in which these sensitized cells perform this function is not understood and this is an important area of current immunological research. This form of immunity is known as cell-mediated immunity.

General features
It is important to note that the immune response is a physio-logical reaction to the introduction into the body of **foreign** material, irrespective of whether it is harmful or not. Further, the

response may be directed at antigens which are inside microorganisms and thus inaccessible to the serum proteins so that they perform no protective role. In contrast to innate immune mechanisms which vary greatly between species, the acquired response is little different between species and the main differences that can be detected occur between individuals.

The genetic control of the immune response

In 1938 Gorer and Schultze showed that there was a correlation between resistance to salmonella infections and the ability to produce antibody. Since this early work a large body of evidence has accumulated showing that the ability of an individual to respond to a particular antigen is under genetic control. There appear to be two forms of this control. (1) Control of the **general capacity** to produce an antibody response. This can be demonstrated by selective breeding of guinea-pigs or mice, which in a few generations can be divided into groups that give a uniformly good or a uniformly poor antibody response to several antigens. The poor response appears likely to be due to the slower mitotic division time of the responding cells. (2) Other genes are able to control the immune response to a **particular antigen** (e.g. a synthetic polypeptide in mice).

The genes controlling the ability to produce an immune response are called **immune response** or **Ir genes** and can be shown to be closely related in their position on a chromosome (number 17 in the mouse) to the genes controlling certain surface antigens of cells. These surface antigens are the major antigenic determinants in graft rejection (see chap. 7, p. 107) and are called histocompatibility antigens.

The discovery of the immune response genes and their close linkage with the major histocompatibility antigen system in several animal species has given considerable impetus in recent years to a search for an association between susceptibility to a variety of neoplastic, autoimmune and infectious diseases and the activity of these genes. These associations are discussed in later chapters (pp. 84 and 148).

Active and passive immunity

An acquired immune state may be brought about in an individual in two main ways: (1) induced by overt clinical infection, inapparent clinical infection or deliberate artificial immunization. This is termed **actively acquired immunity** and contrasts with (2) **passively acquired immunity** which is transferred from an

Table 4.1

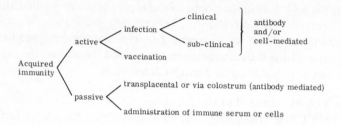

actively immunized individual to a non-immune individual by means of blood, serum components or experimentally by lymphoid cells.

Actively acquired immunity

Actively acquired immunity due to infectious agents fall into two general categories. Some infections, such as diphtheria, whooping cough, smallpox and mumps, usually induce a **lifetime immunity**. Others such as the common cold, influenza, pneumococcal pneumonia and bacillary dysentery, confer immunity for a shorter time, sometimes for only a **few weeks**. Failure of the second group of infections to induce lasting immunity is due to various factors, particularly to the fact that different members or strains of the same species of organism may be involved, and the acquisition of immunity to one strain does not prevent infection by another strain of the same organism.

The role of **nutritional factors** in the acquired immune response has been studied in experimental animals. Of the lymphoid organs the thymus appears to be affected the most, although the other lymphoid organs decrease in weight on severely restricted diets. The red pulp of the spleen and the lymphoid follicles are reduced in size. The absolute number of B lymphocytes are considerably reduced and is reflected in a failure of the lymph nodes to increase in cellularity on antigenic challenge with a consequent reduction particularly in the humoral response. Cell-mediated immunity may be less affected by poor nutrition, particularly in adults, because of the presence of long-lived recirculating lymphocytes (p. 78).

Passively acquired immunity

Administration of immune sera usually prepared in another species, e.g. the horse, is a therapeutic procedure in diphtheria and in gas gangrene. Anti tetanic serum is used prophylactically when wounds may be contaminated with tetanus spores. Passive immunity may be conferred on the infant by the passage of maternal antibody across the **placenta** in some species such as the human and the rabbit, where a particular part of the immunoglobulin polypeptide chain has been found to be necessary for bringing about the transfer process (p. 57). In other species such as the rat and the dog antibodies are also transmitted in the **colostrum** to the intestine. Other animals, notably the lamb and the calf, receive this form of immunity only by means of the colostrum.

Pooled human immunoglobulin is also used as a source of antibody in a number of situations including measles infection and infectious hepatitis, when it is given during the incubation period to modify the attack. Human immunoglobulin is also given to patients with a congenital inability to make antibody globulin (p. 91).

THE TISSUES INVOLVED IN SYNTHESIS OF ANTIBODY

The lymphoid tissues which are predominantly engaged in the immune response are the **lymph nodes, spleen** and **bone marrow.** Whilst the lung and to a lesser extent the liver can both take part in the immune response, their contribution is much less than that of the other tissues. The large overall contribution of the bone marrow is a reflection of the mass of this tissue throughout the skeleton. However, weight for weight the spleen and lymph nodes by far exceed the capacity for antibody production of the bone marrow. For this reason much effort has been expended in attempting to unravel the way in which the specialized lymphoid organs, the spleen and lymph nodes take up foreign antigens and initiate the immune process.

The role of the thymus gland and co-operation between different cell populations in the early events preceding antibody synthesis will be described later in this chapter.

The spleen, lymph nodes, bone marrow and other lymphatic tissues that engage in antibody production are **vascular filtration systems.** They depend on a three dimensional network of reticular cells and reticular fibres. In these filters, **antigen** is **trapped** and **cells** become lodged from the circulating blood and lymph and can **interact, differentiate** and **proliferate** in the organ.

Gross structure

The **lymph nodes** of the human are structures of the shape and approximate size of a bean. In smaller animals they are of the same general structure but correspondingly smaller. The lymph flows

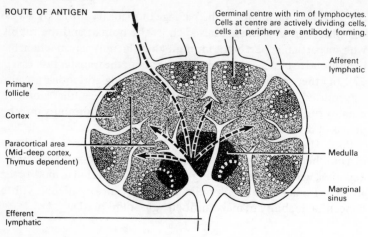

ROUTE OF ANTIGEN ⎯⎯⎯⎯⎯

Germinal centre with rim of lymphocytes.
Cells at centre are actively dividing cells,
cells at periphery are antibody forming.

Afferent
lymphatic

Primary
follicle

Cortex

Paracortical area
(Mid-deep cortex,
Thymus dependent)

Medulla

Marginal
sinus

Efferent
lymphatic

Fig. 4.1 Lymph node

from the limbs and organs through the lymph nodes on its way to
the main lymphatic vessels of the neck and their union with the
veins. The afferent lymphatics enter the capsule of the node (Fig.
4.1) and the lymph leaves via the efferent lymphatics of the hilum.
Trabeculae extend radially into the node from the capsule passing
from the marginal lymph sinus through the cortex to the medulla.
The tissue of the gland consists of a meshwork of reticular cells in
which large numbers of **lymphocytes** are embedded. These cells
are grouped in nodules or **follicles** in the cortex and form
interconnected cords in the medullary area sometimes called
medullary cords. Around each nodule in the cortex is a conden-
sation of reticular cells. A reticular network provides a scaffolding
for the lymphocytes, makes up the sinuses and supports the blood
vessels and nerves. A nodule that enlarges after antigenic
stimulation is termed a **germinal centre** and includes macrophages
with cytoplasmic extensions or dendritic processes. **Macrophages**
are present throughout the gland, many being found in the medullary
area. **Plasma cells** and their precursors are also found particularly
at the cortico-medullary junction. Arteries enter the node at the
hilium and their capillaries end up in post-capillary venules with a
tall lining endothelium. Between and through these endothelial cells
blood lymphocytes pass into the node.

The spleen (Fig. 4.2) like the lymph nodes is enclosed by a capsule
and divided by trabeculae into communicating compartments. The
organ plays an important role in destruction of **red cells** and their
production; as well as producing **platelets**, **granulocytes** and

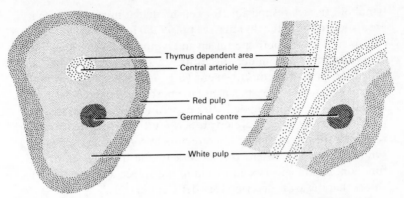

Fig. 4.2 Structure of Malpighian corpuscle. Transverse section of part of spleen showing area of white pulp related to central arteriole and considered to be thymus-dependent.

lymphocytes. Its major immunological role is to act as a filter for the bloodstream. The tissue consists of (a) the **white pulp**–around the branches of the splenic artery which are surrounded by periarterial lymphatic sheaths and lymphatic nodules or Malpighian bodies, and (b) the **red pulp**–splenic sinuses and splenic cords, the latter making up bands of tissue, reticulum cells, erythrocytes, lymphocytes and granulocytes–lying between the sinuses which are themselves lined by 'sinus-lining cells' held together by a network of reticular fibres. The blood leaves the white pulp via capillaries and enters the red pulp passing into the sinuses and is collected up into venules and veins leaving by the splenic vein. The precise details of the blood circulation in the spleen are not yet fully elucidated, but particulate material and cells can clearly pass through the walls of splenic vessels or be discharged directly into the splenic tissue (p. 83). It can thus be seen that the lymph nodes and spleen can be regarded as a complex organization of three types of cell involved in the initiation of the immune reaction–lymphocytes, plasma cells and phagocytic cells of the mono-nuclear phagocyte system.

This account of the structure and histological detail of the spleen and lymph nodes must not obscure the fact that many of the cells in these organs are part of a mobile population circulating between the blood and lymphoid tissues (p. 82).

Development
The lymphoid tissues responsible for humoral antibody production are associated developmentally with the gut and consist of lymphocytes and plasma cells of the lymph node and spleen. The

lymphoid tissues responsible for cell-mediated immune reactivity are associated with the thymus (see pp. 77–80 for further discussion on this subject). In both the spleen and lymph nodes there are areas of lymphoid tissues under the influence of the thymus – the so-called **thymus-dependent areas** (Fig. 4.2)–lying adjacent to the central arterioles in the spleen and the post-capillary venules in the medulla of the lymph node. After experimental neonatal thymec-tomy these areas do not develop properly and cell-mediated immune reactions are absent. There is a rare human condition (Di George's syndrome, p. 90) where this occurs in the absence of thymus function. Histological examination of the spleen and lymph nodes shows that the areas described are deficient in cells.

In the humoral immune response, immunoglobulins are secreted into the blood by lymphoid cells–predominantly **plasma cells** situated in the spleen and lymph nodes. In contrast the cell-mediated response when it occurs peripherally (e.g. in the skin) is effected by migration of the stimulated cells themselves from the lymphoid tissue via the efferent lymphatics to the blood stream, which some of the cells leave through the capillary endothelium to pass into the tissue fluids where they are ready to interact with foreign antigenic material. These cells are then collected by the afferent lymphatics and recirculate.

Organized lymphoid tissues are **absent in invertebrates** and the most primitive of the vertebrates, the hag fish. This system develops late in phylogeny and the first traces appear in the lamprey. Both these primitive vertebrates are, however, able to show a limited degree of adaptive immunity. Their serum contains a primitive form of immunoglobulin that appears to be related to IgM (see below), which has since become considerably diversified. The amphibians are the most primitive animals to show IgG, and all species higher in the evolutionary scale than birds have IgM, IgG and IgA.

The precursors of the early immunoglobulins are likely to have arisen in the prevertebrate era although as yet there is no direct evidence for this. It has been suggested that they may have arisen from receptors on the surface of phagocytes which enable the cells to distinguish foreign material from self. It seems possible that such receptors could have the molecular properties of the combining site of an antibody molecule (see below).

The **complement system** appeared some time later in evolution and is developed in the jawed vertebrate, the paddle fish. With increasing structural complexity of animal species the immune reaction has beome more diversified and effective. However, once components of the immune system appear in evolution they are maintained with a remarkable constancy both at the molecular and functional level.

In the human, lymphoid tissue appears first in the thymus at about eight weeks' gestation. Peyer's patches are distinguishable by the fifth month and immunoglobulin secreting cells appear in the spleen and lymph nodes at about 20 weeks. From this period onwards both IgM and IgG globulins (p. 47) are synthesized by the fetus with IgM predominating. At birth the infant has a blood concentration of IgG comparable to, or sometimes higher than, that of maternal serum having received IgG but not IgM via the placenta from the mother (p. 57). The rate of synthesis of IgM in the infant increases rapidly within the first few days of life but does not reach adult levels until about a year. This compares with the much slower rise in IgG and IgA globulins which do not reach adult levels until between the sixth and seventh years of life. Cell-mediated immune reactions can be stimulated at birth but these reactions (e.g. homegraft rejection) may not be as powerful as in the adult, although the evidence for this is rather scanty.

Invertebrate immunity

For many years it had been generally assumed that the adaptive immune response was a characteristic of the vertebrates and that invertebrates lacked the ability to mount an immune response. The recent recognition of a limited ability in the most primitive of the vertebrates the hag fish to exhibit cell-mediated immunity, suggests that the origins of the immune response may well have been rather earlier. Immunologists are now exploring the possibility that invertebrates can produce at least some form of adaptive immune response.

Specific recognition by certain primitive marine organisms (coelenterates) of the cells of unrelated species is a well-documented phenomenon and can be seen in colonial hydroids, gorgonians and reef-building corals. **Rejection of grafts** shows convincing specificity but no immunological memory leading to accelerated rejection on second exposure, has been demonstrated.

Invertebrates have a well developed **non-specific** cellular defence mechanism to cope with foreign materials that enter its tissues. The process is mediated by blood cells called **haemocytes** which phagocytose the foreign particle and localize it in a fibrous nodule. This process is quite distinct from the cell-mediated immune response of vertebrates as it does not result in the formation of a descendent family or clone of cells with a specificity limited to the

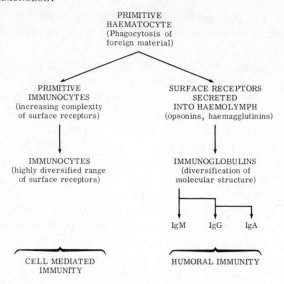

Fig. 4.3 Schematic view of proposed stages in evolutionary development of adaptive immune response.

inducing agent (see Fig. 4.3). Evidence has, however, been obtained in work with annelids and echinoderms showing that they are capable of rejecting grafts from unrelated members of the same species. On repeated grafting **accelerated rejection** takes place indicating the development of what could be a secondary immune response. It seems clear that the mechanism underlying this rejection process is quite distinct from the non-specific haemocyte response to any foreign substance and may well turn out on further study to be a form of specific adaptive immune response.

The tissue fluids of invertebrates have been known for many years to contain a variety of **agglutinins** for vertebrate eythrocytes. These haemagglutinins can be shown to act as **opsonins** (p.56) facilitating phagocytosis. Many attempts have been made unsuccessfully to increase the quantity of these haemagglutinins in the tissue fluids by immunization of invertebrate species (e.g. in cray fish). Of some interest is the finding that the natural haemagglutinin of the horseshoe crab is a protein of molecular weight of approximately 400,000 consisting of 18 subunits of 22,500 each. The subunits have a molecular weight comparable to that of a vertebrate light chain and some similarity in their amino acid composition. These findings have led to the suggestion that the haemagglutinin may represent the product of a primitive form of light chain gene.

Some recent work indicates that certain invertebrate agglutinins are **specific** for cell wall **carbohydrate** determinants, e.g. N-acetyl D galactosamine and N-acetyl neuraminic acid. These findings have potentially important implications for understanding of the evolution of the immunoglobulins of higher animals. The precursor of these was a form of immunoglobulin M found in the most primitive vertebrates. Immunoglobulin M production by B lymphocytes is readily stimulated by carbohydrate antigens and the ability to produce immunoglobulins to non-carbohydrate antigens is probably a much more recently evolved and much more complicated process that requires co-operation between different cells of the lymphoid population.

Cell types resembling vertebrate lymphocytes have been observed in the tissue fluid of annelids but there seems to be considerable doubt that such cells are in fact the precursors of vertebrate lymphoid cells. Lymphocytes do seem to be present in later phyla, the protochordates, as well as macrophages and eosinophils.

The finding of late complement components in invertebrates suggests that the alternate pathway (p. 17) may be phylogenetically more ancient than the classical complement system.

In conclusion it appears that immunological phenomena such as **recognition** and **phagocytosis** are found in the earliest eukaryotic cells. Recognition is responsible for maintenance of **specific partnerships** in metazoa, for exclusion of potentially harmful **microorganisms** and perhaps also for removal of altered or dead tissue constituents. **Cellular immune mechanisms**, such as rejection of unrelated tissue cells (initially without immunological memory), is a feature of all eukaryotic animals and precedes the development of humoral immunity. The emergence of organised lymphoid tissues occurred in the early vertebrate era and immune mechanisms became increasingly efficient with the development of cooperative relationships between the different cellular elements.

THE IMMUNE RESPONSE

Immunoglobulin production—the humoral antibody response

The antibody response resulting from exposure to antigenic substances has certain well defined characteristics. After first meeting the antigen there is an interval of about two weeks before antibody can be found in the blood, and during this initial period there is intense activity in the antibody-forming tissues. This can be shown by studies with isotope-labelled precursors of cell components, for example tritiated thymidine, to show DNA synthesis or carbon-14 labelled amino acids in protein synthesis. Following antigenic stimulation there is a rapid increase in cell proliferation and synthesis of protein in the cells of the lymphoid organs indicated by the incorporation of the labelled materials. If the lymphoid cell population of a rat is depleted, by placing a cannula in the thoracic duct and the lymph is drained off, then no such cell proliferation takes place and there is no antibody response. In contrast in a normal animal immunized for instance with sheep red blood cells, lymphocytes taken from the spleen or lymph nodes can be shown to have synthesized anti-sheep cell antibodies because if sheep red cells are mixed with the spleen or lymph gland cells the red cells aggregate around individual lymphocytes giving a rosette appearance when examined microscopically (Fig. 4.4). The red cells become attached to the surface of lymphocytes by means of antibody located at the cell membrane.

The antibody which eventually can be detected in the blood – the so-called **primary immune response** does not reach a high level and does not persist unless a second dose of antigen is given (Fig. 4.5). When this happens, any remaining antibody will be rapidly mopped up by combination with the antigen and this will be reflected by a fall in detectable antibody in the blood; then after only a day or two a remarkable rise in the level of antibody begins and reaches a peak shortly thereafter which can be from 10 to 50 times higher than the primary response. This **secondary response** is mainted at a high level falling only slowly over a period of months. The response can be boosted to even higher levels by further injections of antigen until a stage is reached when no further increase occurs. It is important to note that once an animal has responded to an antigen, even though exposed to it on only one occasion, the animal retains a **memory** of the antigen so that even after an interval of months or years it is able to react by means of a secondary response with a rapid mobilization of antibody-forming cells. Hence vaccination against an infective agent such as smallpox or poliomyelitis virus provides many years of useful protection against infection, even though soon after vaccination the level of antibodies falls to a low level, since the memory has been retained.

To obtain a maximum response, the **interval** between the primary and secondary injections should not be too short and an interval of less than 10 days is likely to reduce the level of the secondary response; subsequent injections should be spaced out to weeks then to months (p. 69). This allows time for the increase in numbers of antibody-forming cells which can be stimulated by

IMMUNO-CYTO-ADHERENCE
Rosette technique

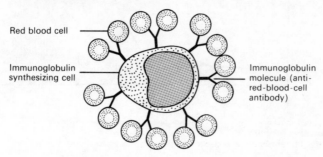

Red blood cell

Immunoglobulin
synthesizing cell

Immunoglobulin
molecule (anti-
red-blood-cell
antibody)

LOCALISED HAEMOLYSIS IN GEL
Jerne Plaque technique

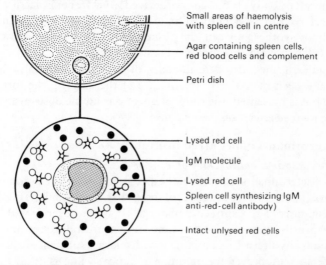

Small areas of haemolysis
with spleen cell in centre

Agar containing spleen cells,
red blood cells and complement

Petri dish

Lysed red cell

IgM molecule

Lysed red cell

Spleen cell synthesizing IgM
anti-red-cell antibody)

Intact unlysed red cells

Fig. 4.4 Two methods for demonstrating antibody formation by single cells. In the immuno-cyto-adherence test spleen cells from an animal immunized with, for example, sheep red blood cells, are mixed with the red cell antigen and after a period of incubation 'rosettes' are formed as shown. The red cells often completely surround the antibody-producing spleen cells. In the Jerne plaque technique, the spleen cells from the sheep-cell immunized animal are mixed with the red cell antigen in soft agar and when complement (guinea-pig serum) is layered on the surface, lysis of the red cells occurs. This happens because the antibody produced by the spleen cell has diffused into the surrounding agar and coated the red cells. This enables the complement system to be activated with the resulting lysis of the red cell (see p. 16 for the description of complement lysis).

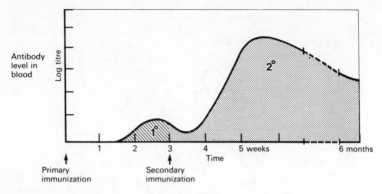

Fig. 4.5 The antibody response

subsequent injections. The lymphocytes engaged in the initiation of humoral antibody production are derived from the bone marrow and are referred to as **B cells**. This cell differentiates into the main antibody synthesizing cell–the **plasma cell**. The characteristics of this cell population are discussed later in this chapter.

Some of the host determinants of acquired immunity have already been mentioned. The nature of the antigen, the form in which it is presented, the route of injection and the dose given also have marked effects on the response.

Determinants of acquired immunity

Form, dose and route of entry of antigen
The determinants of antigenic specificity have been discussed above (p. 21), as have the effect of molecular weight and the need for foreignness of the antigenic material. It is, however, possible to enhance the natural ability of an antigen to induce an immune response by altering it or mixing it with another substance (called an adjuvant). A procedure of much practical value is to alter the **physical state** of the antigen by adsorbing it on to mineral gels such as aluminium hydroxide or phosphate. These alum-precipitated antigens are widely used as immunizing agents for humans. Such particulate forms of antigens seem to be able to initiate antibody production much more effectively than the same antigens in non-particulate form. This effect is not fully understood but may be due to a direct effect of the particulate material on the lymphocyte cell membrane leading to more effective transformation of the cell for antibody formation than can be brought about by antigen in solution. An additional factor which may be important for some types of antigen is that particulate material is more readily phagocytosed by

macrophages. These cells have been shown in certain situations to make a contribution by serving as a store of antigen for later release and stimulation of lymphocytes. It has been suggested that macrophages may also improve the antigenicity of weak antigens by altering them in some way before passing them on to lymphocytes. It is conceivable also that by removing antigen from the circulation they protect the lymphocytes from the effects of excess antigen which would be likely to paralyse the lymphocytes rather than initiate antibody production (p. 64). For a protein antigen a dose of a few hundred microgrammes is required to stimulate the production of detectable circulating antibody. The increase in antibody response is small in proportion to the increase in dose of antigen given and is approximately proportional to the square root of the increase in antigen administered until an upper limit is reached. An increase above this level can, as indicated above, result in specific paralysis of the antibody-forming tissues. This form of inhibition, sometimes referred to as **immunological tolerance** is specific only for the antigen which brought it about. The lymphoid tissues remain normally responsive to other antigens.

Other methods have been developed to enhance the antibody response, although at present they are used mainly in experimental work. The most important of these consists of the preparation of a **water-in-oil emulsion** (Fig. 4.6): an aqueous solution of antigen is emulsified in a light mineral oil so that tiny drops of antigen solution are dispersed throughout the oil. The emulsion forms a depot of antigen in the subcutaneous tissues from which small quantities of antigen are continually released, sometimes for a year or more. An influenza vaccine in this form has been used successfully in man.

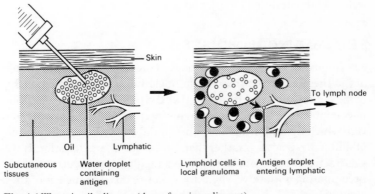

Skin

To lymph node

Oil   Lymphatic

Subcutaneous tissues

Water droplet containing antigen

Lymphoid cells in local granuloma

Antigen droplet entering lymphatic

Fig. 4.6 Water in oil adjuvant (depot forming adjuvant)

New possibilities have been opened up by the development in Edinburgh of a multiple form of emulsion, in which the aqueous solution is first dispersed in oil and the oil is finally dispersed in a water phase. These emulsions are stable and much less viscous and less difficult to inject that the water-in-oil type. An even better response is achieved if killed tubercle bacilli are included in the emulsion; a wax constituent of the bacterial wall is responsible for this effect. The bacterial product appears to stimulate .the cells involved in the immune response. Such emulsions are of course suitable for experimental work and are often termed **Freund's** adjuvants after their originator.

The advantages of these **adjuvant** methods of immunization are that both the primary and secondary immune response are achieved by only one injection of antigen and that the peak level of antibody is maintained over a long period by the small quantities of antigen released from the depot.

Table 4.2 gives a list of examples of the three main types of adjuvant that are used **depot** or **repository, bacterial** and **chemical.** The main effects of these adjuvants on the immune system (where known) are shown in the table. In the last few years adjuvants have been widely employed in tumour immunotherapy, both in experimental animals and man, and this is discussed further on page 170.

If an antigen is given intravenously most of the antibody is produced by the spleen, and some in the lung and bone marrow; on the other hand, if given subcutaneously or intradermally, the antigen travels via lymphatics to the local lymph nodes where antibody production is initiated. When antigen is given with adjuvants, there is a local accumulation of inflammatory cells, and antibody production occurs in the resulting granulomatous tissue as well as in the draining lymph nodes.

THE IMMUNOGLOBULINS

Enormous advances have been made in the last decade in knowledge of the chemical structure of immunoglobulins and the relationship of the **structure** to the **biological activities** of the molecule. These have enabled immunologists to agree internationally on a nomenclature which distinguishes a number of different classes of immunoglobulin on structural rather than functional characteristics. It was the practice to refer to an antibody as an agglutinin, a neutralizing or a precipitating antibody, when it was not realized that each of these activities could be exhibited by a chemically heterogeneous

Table 4.2 Adjuvants

Type	Example	Main effects
Depot or repository		
Aluminium and calcium compounds	Aluminium phosphate	Slow release of antigen and local granuloma
Water in oil emulsions of antigen	Freund's incomplete	Slow release of antigen, emulsion droplets carry antigen to lymph nodes, local granuloma
Bacterial		
Mycobacteria	BCG (sometimes in water in oil emulsion – Freund's complete)	Stimulation of macrophage activity, increases numbers of antibody-producing cells
Anaerobic coryneforms	Corynebacterium parvum	Stimulation of macrophage activity, augmentation of certain classes of immunoglobulin e.g. IgM. Immunostimulation for antibody responses and immunosuppression of cell-mediated immune responsiveness.
Bordetella	B. pertussis	Activation of macrophages, lymphocytosis (shift of lymphocytes from T and B cell areas of lymphoid tissues)
Bacterial polysaccharides	various gram –ve organisms	Activation of lymphocytes
Chemical		
Lysolecithin analogues	C_{18} ether hydroxy lysolecithin	Activation of macrophages
Lysozome labilizers	Vitamin A, beryllium salts silica	Activation of macrophages
Polyanions	Double stranded, natural and synthetic polyribonucleic acids	Increase numbers of memory cells, activation of T lymphocytes and macrophages (interferon production)
Fungal polysaccharides	Lentinan (a glucose polymer)	Not known (possible stimulation of T lymphocytes)
Imidazole derivative	Levamisole	Not known

population of molecules and could be shared by the same molecule. Other classifications were dependent on the behaviour of the molecules in electrophoresis, which did little more than split the population up into still heterogeneous groups of proteins differing in their overall charge and molecular size.

Methods have been developed in America for the fragmentation of the immunoglobulin molecule by chemical cleavage in Edelman's laboratory, and by pepsin digestion by Nisonoff. Porter in Britain was the first to achieve cleavage with retention of biological activity of the fragments using papain digestion. These studies gave impetus to the work which now has enabled immunologists to distinguish five main classes of immunoglobulin each based on a similar polypeptide chain structure consisting of two pairs of 'heavy' and 'light' chains joined by disulphide bonds sometimes occurring as multiples of this basic unit.

It is considered that the molecule is based on a **12-unit structure**, each unit consisting of a polypeptide chain with 110 amino acids of MW 12,000. Each light chain of MW 25,000 consists of two of the basic units and each heavy chain four basic units. Heterogeneity of immunoglobulin structure occurs within this general framework with some of the basic units being affected more than others. Figure 4.7 shows a tentative view of how the molecule may have evolved from the basic unit, perhaps arising as a receptor on a phagocytic cell. The evolutionary advantage provided by antibody-like molecules has ensured their maintenance and diversification over hundreds of millions of years. A picture of the immunoglobulin molecule has

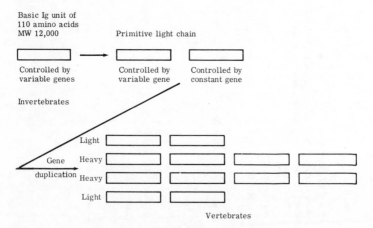

Fig. 4.7 Possible evolution of the immunoglobulin molecule.

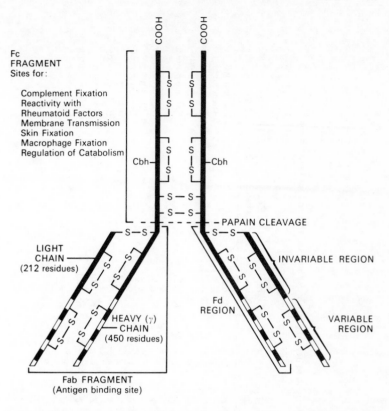

Fig. 4.8 Diagrammatic view of structural arrangements of polypeptide chains of immunoglobulin molecule. The chains are held together by three disulphide bonds. Pepsin splits the molecule, leaving an Fc fragment (crystallizable) and Fd parts of the heavy chains with attached light chains – the whole making Fab (or antigen binding) fragments. The N terminal ends of the light and heavy chains have variable sequences of amino acids as shown by the broken line. There are also a number of intra-chain disulphide bonds which influence the shape of individual chains. The carbohydrate (Cbh) groups may be concerned with the catabolism of the molecule.

been built up and is represented in Figure 4.8. The general arrangement has been confirmed by electron microscopy.

On the basis of marked **antigenic differences** in the **heavy chains** it has been possible to define **five classes** of human immunoglobulin, using the technique of immunoelectrophoresis. These are referred to as IgG, IgM, IgA, IgE and IgD (Table 4.3) (Fig. 4.9). IgM seems to have been the first immunoglobulin molecule to evolve. IgG and IgA probably evolved from the IgM by loss of a single basic unit (domain) from the heavy chains (see below).

Table 4.3 Human immunoglobulins (Levels vary widely, males tend to have slightly lower levels of IgG and IgM but higher IgA)

Immunoglobulin class	Serum concentration mg/100 ml	Molecular weight	Half life days	Light chains	Heavy chains	Characteristic properties
IgG	900–1800	160,000	18–23	K and L	γ	Precipitins Antitoxins Complement fixation Late antibody
IgA	156–294	170,000 and polymers	5–6.5	K and L	α	Surface protection
IgM	67–145	960,000	5	K and L	μ	Agglutinins Opsonins Lysins, complement fixation Early antibody
IgD	0.3–40	184,000	2.8	K and L	δ	Not known
IgE	10–130 (μg)	188,105	2.3	K and L	ε	Reaginic antibody

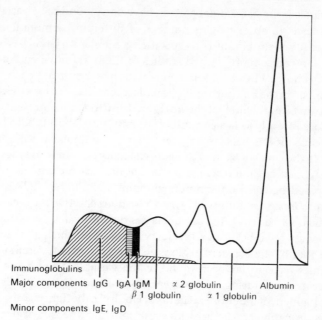

Immunoglobulins
Major components IgG IgA IgM   α 2 globulin   Albumin
                   β 1 globulin   α 1 globulin
Minor components IgE, IgD

Fig. 4.9 Electrophoretogram obtained by UV scanning of paper electrophoresis strip and showing diagrammatically the main components of human serum and the immunoglobulin classes.-

Immunoglobulin G or IgG

This is the major immunoglobulin component of serum making up 75 per cent of the total and having a molecular weight of 160,000 in the human. The molecule has two antigen-binding sites as shown in Figure 4.8 on what are termed the **Fab** portions of the molecule and involving part of both the heavy and light chains. The amino acid sequences have been worked out in whole or in part for a small number of light and heavy chains in various species, using myeloma proteins which are present as a homogeneous population in the serum of individuals with plasma cell tumours in sufficient quantity to enable studies of this type to be made.

The light chains can be shown to consist of two parts joined together. One has a **constant** sequence of amino acids at the C terminal end of the chain, common to the light chains of the species under study. The other part is at the N terminal end in which **variation** occurs in the sequence of the 107 amino acids. The variable portion differs between one myeloma and another, being similar only within a particular myeloma. Up to 50 per cent of the positions in the N terminal portion have been found to be variable. This leads to an enormous number of different permutations of sequence and thus in antibody specificity. Similar variation has been found in rather more limited studies of the N terminal end of the **heavy chain**. The variable portions of the light and heavy chains are contained in the Fab portion of the molecule and it is in this **variable portion** of the chain that the **antigen-binding** site is present.

More recently as larger numbers of immunoglobulins have been sequenced it has become apparent that the amino acid variability tends to be concentrated in three so-called **hypervariable** regions. The remaining amino acid sequences of the variable regions, when compared between one immunoglobulin and another, fall into V region subclasses (four for K chain V regions and five for L chain).

The discovery of V region subclasses demonstrates that V region sequences have been more **strictly conserved** during evolution than that of the constant regions. No species specific amino acid residues have so far been found in the variable portion and this suggests that during embryogenesis a single gene controls the development of the entire range of variability in the light chains. This gene probably arose early in evolution and the survival value associated with diversification of the antigen-binding site has ensured its maintenance since then.

The **light chains** are of two distinct types known as K or L (κ or λ) chains. In any one individual, both K and L chains are produced but they are not found together in the same immunoglobulin molecule. K and L chains are present in a ratio of about 2:1 in any one individual. Two intra-chain disulphide bonds (Fig. 4.8) occur in almost exactly the same position in both K and L chains and both chains have cysteine as the terminal amino acid at the carboxyl end. This serves for the attachment to the heavy chains. These facts suggest a **common genetic origin** of K and L chains which, although they have **diverged** during evolution, have retained many common structural characteristics.

The **heavy chains** are specific for each class; in the human IgG molecule the heavy chain or γ chain exists in four different forms, IgG1, IgG2, IgG3 and IgG4, which can be distinguished by specific antisera able to detect differences in the Fc fragment of the heavy chains. Sixty-five per cent of the IgG molecules in human serum are of the IgG subclass, 23 per cent of the IgG2 and 8 per cent and 4 per cent IgG3 and 4. Differences have been found in the numbers and position of the disulphide bonds in the different IgG subclasses and these are shown diagrammatically in Fig. 4.10. Disulphide bonds are essential to the normal 3-dimensional

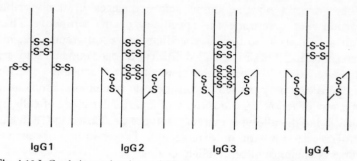

IgG1   IgG2   IgG3   IgG4

Fig. 4.10 IgG subclasses showing variable arrangements of the disulphide bonds.

structure of immunoglobulin molecules and differences in their location may be reflected in different biological activities.

The separate immunoglobulin chains consist of repeating homologous units called **domains**; two for light chains, four or five for heavy chains (μ and ε heavy chains have five). A so-called 'hinge' region occurs on heavy chains of all classes except IgM. It is inserted between the Fd and Fc portions and contains the inter heavy chain disulphide bridges.

The domains show many **homologies** in their amino acid sequences and were probably derived from an ancestral gene coding for the length of one domain. This gene was presumably doubled then redoubled and, within each resulting gene, crossing-over and mutation has since led to the differences that can now be detected in their products. The further back in evolution that divergence between the genes took place, the fewer the similarities. The generation of subclasses is relatively recent in evolution and there is therefore a high degree of homology.

Individuals can be subdivided on the basis of certain characteristics of their immunoglobulin molecules. These are comparable to the blood groups but instead of involving antigenic differences in the surface antigens of red cells, they depend on antigenic differences in the light and heavy chains of the immunoglobulin molecule. These genetically determined sub-groups are known as **allotypes**. Three main groups, Gm, Km and Am, have been found and each can be subdivided. The antigenic determinants of the Gm groups are carried in the γ chains of the IgG molecule only. In contrast the Km factors are present in the K light chains of each of the immunoglobulin classes. Am allotypes have been found in the IgA2 subclass.

The variable portions of the heavy and light chains of the Fab fragment have also been shown to carry antigenic determinants.

These depend on the amino acid sequences in the variable portion that determine the specificity of the antibody. Thus Fab fragments of different specificity have different antigenic determinants. These are called **idiotypic** determinants and are characteristic of the particular clone of cells producing a specific antibody and have proved of considerable value to immunologists as a way of following the activity of a particular clone of cells by identifying the idiotypic marker. Isotypes also exist and are due to antigenic determinants on all molecules of a certain class or subclass of heavy chains or of certain light chains.

IgM, IgA and IgD
Like IgG globulin each of these classes of immunoglobulin in man has been found to contain K and L light chains. The heavy chains, on the other hand, are unique for each of these types of immunoglobulin, IgM containing μ chains. μ chains have five subunits or domains (one variable and four constant) compared with four subunits in γ and α heavy chains. IgE (see p. 96), like IgM, also has an extra domain in its ε heavy chain. IgA have α chains and IgD δ chains and it is these differences which enable them to be distinguished one from another. There are two subclasses of IgA (IgA1 and IgA2). IgA2 is unusual in that the light chains are linked to each other by disulphide bonds instead of to the heavy chains (they are linked covalently to the heavy chains in this subclass) IgA1 accounts for 90 per cent of the total serum IgA in contrast to secretions, where IgA2 makes up as much as 60 per cent of the total. IgM globulin with a molecular weight of about 900,000 can be split by reduction of disulphide bonds into five subunits. These subunits have a molecular weight of 180,000 and are believed like IgG to have two heavy and two light chains.

Until recently most studies on the number of antigen-binding sites of IgM antibody showed that the molecule had only five binding sites despite the fact that theoretically 10 were present. Both human and rabbit IgM however have now been shown to have the 10 sites and it is believed that the two binding sites on each are unable to combine with antigen with similar efficiency thus making it difficult to demonstrate all 10 sites. Polymeric forms of IgA and the IgM molecule have recently been shown to have a small polypeptide called the J chain.

This polypeptide has a molecular weight of about 15,000 and differs in structure from all known immunoglobulin polypeptide chains. It is rich in cysteine residues and appears to exist in a molar ratio of one J chain per polymer regardless of how many immunoglobulin subunits make up the polymer. The J chain makes up about 1 per cent of the IgM molecule by weight and in the IgA molecule about 3 per cent.

The role of the J chain is not entirely clear but the fact that it is added at the final polymerization stage just before the molecule is secreted at the cell membrane of the synthesizing cell suggests that it may be required in the secretion process. It is noteworthy that IgM subunits are not found free in the serum, although polymers of IgM without J chain are found in certain pathological conditions. The role of the J chain in the IgA molecule may be to activate the transport molecules that carry IgA through the mucous membranes and may perhaps be responsible for the ability of the IgA molecule to bind secretory piece (see p. 57). The molecular structure of some of these immunoglobulins is shown in Figures 4.11 and 4.12.

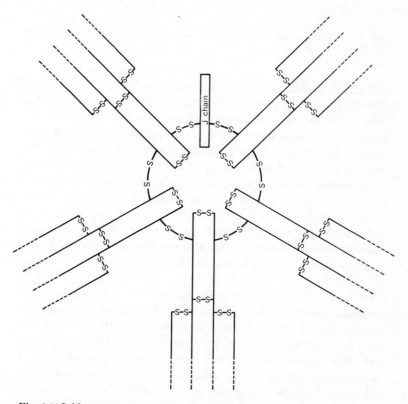

Fig. 4.11 IgM structure showing five subunits and multiple combining sites.

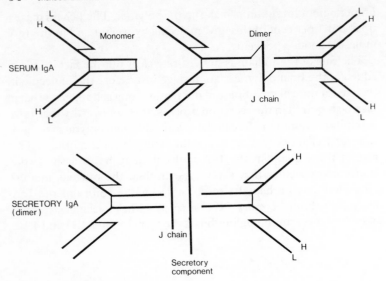

Fig. 4.12 IgA showing monomer, dimer and secretory form, with J chain and secretory component.

Structure and function of immunoglobulins

Knowledge gained from the structural studies discussed above has helped towards an understanding of the biological activities of the immunoglobulin molecule and it is now possible to pinpoint areas of the molecule responsible for different activities. The areas of the light and heavy chains (Fab portion) containing the variable sequences are the site of that part of the molecule with the capacity to combine with antigen. The heavy chain component (Fd portion) seems in some studies to contain as much as 85 per cent of the antigen-binding ability although this is not always so. The light chain component although usually inactive alone seems to act together with the heavy chain to form a stable antigen-binding site.

Complement activation and agglutination. The Fc portion of the molecule appears in IgG molecules to be the major component responsible for activating the complement system, although this does not occur unless two or more molecules of IgG are brought into close apposition. It is not certain exactly what changes in molecular configuration or other effects take place when the molecules come close together but isolated Fc fragments do not activate complement and will do so only if aggregated first. One suggestion is shown in Figure 4.13 in which IgG that has not

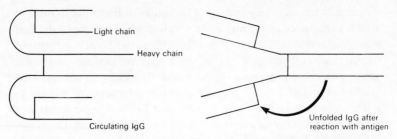

Light chain

Heavy chain

Circulating IgG

Unfolded IgG after
reaction with antigen

Fig. 4.13 Possible molecular forms of IgG before and after combination with antigen (see text).

combined with antigen is represented as folded so that the Fc portion is partly hidden. On combination with antigen the molecule springs open at the hinge region thus exposing the Fc portion which can then activate complement. The subclasses of IgG (Fig. 4.10) vary in their ability to bind complement components, IgG3 appears to bind C1q seven times more effectively than IgG1 and IgG4 does not bind complement at all.

It has been calculated that a single IgM molecule attached to a red cell by its multiple combining sites can bring about lysis whereas 1000 IgG molecules are required for the same effect. Humphrey and Dourmashkin who came to these conclusions assume that as two IgG molecules must come together for complement activation, a large number of IgG molecules would be required for this to occur as the antigenic determinants are spread evenly over the surface of the red cell. Agglutination is brought about by the linking of particulate antigens such as red cells or bacteria by the two Fab fragments of the immunoglobulin molecule. As might be expected from knowledge of the structure of the IgM molecule its five combining sites make it a very efficient agglutinating antibody molecule and rabbit IgM antibacterial antibody is known to be 22 times as active as IgG antibody (mol/mol) in bringing about bacterial agglutination. Because of its large molecular size IgM is largely confined to the blood stream and probably plays an important role in protection. Deficiency of IgM is often associated with susceptibility to septicaemia. IgG antibodies on the other hand are more effective than IgM antibodies at neutralizing diphtheria toxin, lysozyme or viruses such as poliovirus. Whilst some of this activity was present in isolated Fab fragments the evidence from virus neutralization indicates that the Fc fragment may assist the Fab fragments in neutralization of virus infectivity. The molecular basis for such effects has yet to be elucidated.

Tissue fixation and opsonization. The ability of immunoglobulin to attach to tissue cells appears to be a well marked feature of the IgE class of immunoglobulin responsible in humans for various forms of hypersensitivity reaction (p. 96) and may be dependent on the activity of the Fc portion of the molecule. This is suggested by studies of the ability of immunoglobulin fragments to adhere to guinea-pig skin and produce a particular form of hypersensitivity reaction that is known as passive cutaneous anaphylaxis. Immunoglobulin antibody specific for particulate antigens such as bacteria plays a valuable role by coating the surface and making the antigen more susceptible to phagocytosis. These are known as opsonizing antibodies and IgM antibodies perform this role particularly efficiently. In the rabbit it has been shown that IgM anti-salmonella antibodies are some 500 to 1000 times more effective than IgG antibodies as opsonizing agents. How opsonization is brought about is not clear; it is possible that antibody may alter the surface properties, such as the surface charge of a particulate antigen, and thus perhaps reduce electrostatic repulsion between phagocyte and antigen. It also can be shown that the Fc fragments of the antibody have an affinity for the surface of the macrophage and thus link the particulate antigen (attached by means of the antibody combining sites) to the macrophage (attached by the Fc fragment). Antibody with the ability to attach to macrophages by means of the Fc fragment has been described in the guinea-pig and is known as cytophilic antibody. Antigen-antibody complexes appear to be localized in the lymphoid follicles of lymph glands due to the activity of the Fc portion of the immunoglobulin molecule.

The presence of immunoglobulin molecules as receptors for antigen on the surface of lymphocytes has been confirmed by a variety of techniques. B lymphocytes can clearly be shown to have light chains and heavy (μ) chains on their surface, but the situation as far as T cells are concerned is less clear (see p. 81).

Recent work indicates that IgD is present on the majority of B lymphocytes in the cord blood of human infants and in a lesser proportion of adult B lymphocytes. The molecule does not cross the placenta and is absent from cord serum. The significance of these observations is not yet clear. A similar immunoglobulin has been found in the mouse and occurs together with other classes of immunoglobulin on a substantial proportion of B cells in the spleen, lymph nodes and peyers patches. Immature B cells (uncommitted) appear to have μ (IgM) heavy chains and later to develop δ (IgD) chains in addition. At a later stage in differentiation δ and γ (IgG) chains are formed without μ chains.

Selective transport. The newborn animal emerging from an environment where it has been sheltered from antigenic stimuli is protected by maternal immunoglobulins transmitted from the mother. These antibodies often reach a level higher than in the mother and persist longer in the circulation of the young animal than they would do in the adult. This transferred **passive immunity** tides the infant over the period until its own immunological system begins to mature.

In humans, IgG globulins can pass through the placenta and reach the fetal circulation; this is not a simple filtration process, but is due to selective transfer of the molecules involving a part of the Fc fragment of IgG heavy chains. This property is a feature only of the γ heavy chains of IgG and has not been found in the μ and α chains of IgM and IgA. This mechanism seems to be limited to **primates** whilst in **ruminants** maternal immunoglobulins from the colostrum reach the fetus through the intestinal epithelium.

Another selective transport mechanism is found with IgA globulins which are selectively secreted into saliva and respiratory and intestinal **mucous secretions** as well as into the **colostrum**. The site of synthesis of IgA is in submucosal plasma cells of the **lamina propria** of the gastrointestinal tract and in the salivary glands and mammary glands. In the lamina propria of human gastrointestinal tract the IgA producing cells outnumber the IgG cells by about 20:1 in contrast to lymph nodes and spleen where the ratio is 1:3 (IgA:IgG). The IgA found in mucous secretions is manufactured as a dimer with a J chain component and has an attached **secretory** or transport piece not found except in small amounts in serum IgA. It seems likely that it is added to the molecule during its passage into the mucous secretions from the lamina propria, underlying the mucous membrane of the gut and respiratory tract. The secretory component has a molecular weight of 70,000, the J chain 15,000 and the secretory IgA is an 11 S molecule of molecular weight 400,000. The IgM present in secretions has also been found to have secretory component bound to it, whilst any IgG or IgE found in secretions does not. About 4 per cent of the plasma cells of the respiratory and gastrointestinal mucosa are making IgE and, like IgA producing cells, contribute to serum IgE levels.

Salivary and colostral IgA, probably because of the attached secretory piece, appears to be relatively resistant to digestion by proteolytic enzymes in contrast to other immunoglobulins and this would clearly be an advantage in allowing this immuno-globulin to remain active and able to perform a protective role in the intestinal tract. The dimer form of IgA gains the ability to fix complement and after attaching to Gram-negative organisms there is evidence that the activation of the complement system by the IgA may allow the enzyme lysozyme (p. 11) to digest the mucopolysaccharides of the microorganism's cell wall. Much effort is being expended by laboratory workers in studying the role of IgA as a protective mechanism at the mucous surface and the possible future use of vaccines designed to stimulate this form of antibody response may be of considerable value.

An interesting suggestion has been made, supported by some experimental evidence, that IgA in the mucous secretions may inhibit the binding of potentially pathogenic microorganisms to the mucous membranes and thus prevent infection. IgA may play a role by combining with food constituents that could act as allergens and prevent their passage through the gut wall. This idea is supported by the finding that infants with reduced serum IgA levels soon after birth seem more likely to develop allergic states at about 1 year of age. See page 122 for further discussion of IgA activity.

THE CELLS CONCERNED IN
ANTIBODY PRODUCTION

Antigen localization and contact with macrophages and lymphocytes
A simplified picture of the cellular mechanisms leading to antibody formation is that antibodies of different specificities are made by different families or **clones** of cells, each family being genetically programmed to make antibody of only **one specificity**. There is evidence to show that the cells carry at least part of the molecule of their particular antibody exposed on the cell membrane as a receptor for antigen. Thus when an antigen is injected into the body and comes in contact with lymphoid cells it combines with those exposed antibody receptors which are best able to fit the determinant groups of the antigen molecule.

The way this is brought about can be seen when isotope-labelled antigen is injected into an animal, when it is first rapidly localized in the sinus-lining macrophages in the marginal zone around the Malpighian bodies in the spleen or the medullary macrophages of the lymph nodes (Fig. 4.1), depending on the route of injection (p. 42). After this localization, plasma cell precursors (probably small lymphocytes) at the cortico-medullary junction of the lymph nodes are triggered to proliferate and differentiate into antibody-producing cells; exactly how this triggering mechanism works is not yet understood. One possibility is that after partial degradation in the macrophage, antigenic fragments are passed on to the lymphocytes. It is also possible that some antigens can react directly with the lymphocytes themselves (see below). This stimulation and proliferation lead to the development of lymphoid follicles, which are localized collections of active lymphoid cells taking part in the primary immune response.

Subsequent contact with antigen now results in a rather different pattern of localization influenced by the presence of secreted antibody to the antigen; antigen, whilst still taken up by medullary macrophages, is also localized on the surface of **dendritic macrophages** (macrophages with cytoplasmic extensions) which interdigitate with each other and with the lymphoid cells of the lymphoid follicles or Malpighian bodies. This localization seems to depend on antibody at the surface of the macrophage. Lymphocytes themselves may also come directly in contact with antigen. They can be shown to have at least portions of the immunoglobulin molecule on their surface because they can readily be stimulated to respond by transformation, to contact with antibodies directed at various parts of the immunoglobulin molecule. The specificity of these surface immunoglobulins is thought to be determined by the **genetic constitution** of the particular lymphocyte. Nossal in Australia was able to isolate single antibody producing cells in a 'micro droplet' and show that such cells taken from an animal immunized with salmonella produced only one type of antibody. It has been inferred from this that the cell receptor and the secreted antibody are of the same specificity and it has been found that receptors can only be seen clearly on the antibody secreting cell population (i.e. the B cells).

Immunoglobulin heavy chains are present as a component of the immunoglobulin receptor on B cells; they are μ chains as found in IgM and the molecule appears to be an IgM subunit (similar in MW to IgG and called IgMs). B lymphocytes prior to antigenic stimulation are believed to synthesize around 250 to 500 subunits of IgM per hour per cell. The molecules are shed from the surface membrane into the extracellular fluid.

The B cell membrane possesses **receptors** for the Fc fragment of the immunoglobulin molecule and a receptor for the activated complement component C3. It is not yet clear what role these receptors play in B cell activity. The possibility has been suggested that binding of activated C3 leads to B cell activation and that the Fc receptor acts as a receptor site for IgM molecules, in particular subunits of IgM (IgMs), which appear to be the predominant immunoglobulin present on B cells. Another suggestion, based on the ability of antisera directed against histocompatibility antigens to block uptake of labelled complexes of antibody and antigen, is that the Fc receptor is related to the product of the immune response (Ir) genes and that the receptor may be involved in the genetic control of immune responsiveness by B cells. The detailed mechanism underlying these proposals are as yet far from being resolved and await a much clearer understanding of the histocompatibility gene complex and its products as represented in the cell membrane.

Microscopic examination of lymphocytes exposed to antigen has shown that antigen tends to bind preferentially to certain areas of the lymphocyte membrane rather than uniformly over the cell surface. The surface immunoglobulin receptors seem to be able to **coalesce** at points around the cell membrane suggesting that they have a degree of mobility. This finding is consistent with current views on the structure of cell membranes indicating that they are made up of a lipid bilayer containing protein molecules that can move around, coalesce and separate when for example the pH of the surrounding medium is changed.

Properties of antigen, cell co-operation and activation of lymphocytes
Binding of antigen to the immunoglobulin receptors on a B lymphocyte, whilst a necessary prelude to activation of the cell for immunoglobulin synthesis, is not in itself sufficient to ensure B cell stimulation. For successful activation the antigen molecule must have additional properties, rather like the mitogenic properties of phytohaemagglutin (see p. 73), which provide a '**signal**' to activate the cell.

Certain antigens, e.g. bacterial lipopolysaccharides, have this property and can stimulate B cells unaided. Other antigens, e.g. serum proteins, although able to bind to the B cell, are unable to deliver the activating 'signal'. These latter antigens require the assistance of T lymphocytes to **co-operate** with the B lymphocyte and provide the necessary stimulus for activation.

The observations that led to these conclusions allowed the identification of two categories of antigen: (1) those that bind and activate B lymphocytes without the assistance of T lymphocytes, referred to as **T-independent antigens**, and (2) those that can bind to B lymphocytes but require the co-operation of T lymphocytes for B cell activation, referred to as **T-dependent antigens** (Fig. 4.14).

A number of hypotheses have been put forward to explain how B cell stimulation is achieved; they fall into two categories – the so-called '**one signal**' and '**two signal**' models. One signal models propose that B cells can be triggered by antigens with repeating

T independent antigen   T dependent antigen

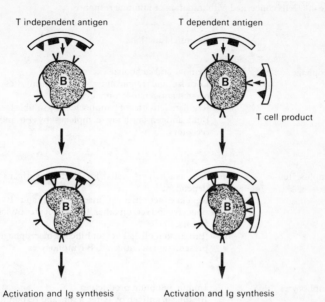

T cell product

Activation and Ig synthesis   Activation and Ig synthesis

Fig. 4.14 Scheme showing how T-independent and T-dependent antigens trigger B lymphocytes to synthesize antibody. Macrophage products may be responsible for activating T lymphocytes (see p. 73) and macrophages themselves may present antigen to B cells (not shown in diagram).

antigenic determinants that cross-link adjacent immunoglobulin receptors on B cells. The T cell in this model is believed to function as a regulator of B cell function—**suppressing** or **stimulating** according to the needs of the situation. Two signal models propose that two specific signals must be delivered to the B cell in order for triggering to occur. Signal 1 is delivered by binding of antigen to the immunoglobulin receptor on the B cell, and Signal 2 by a T cell product or perhaps by a macrophage product (see below). One proposal by Feldman is that the T cell produces a specific immunoglobulin in response to part of the antigen molecule (carrier portion) and that this immunoglobulin (IgT) is cytophilic (i.e. binds) for macrophages. The macrophages then bind antigen and present it to B cells leading to triggering and antibody formation. Direct presentation of antigen to B cells by T lymphocytes has been proposed, perhaps in the form of antigen bridging between the two cells. The T cell binding antigen by receptors that recognize determinants on the protein molecule, itself carries within it smaller (haptenic) determinant groups with which B cells can interact (but not respond to without T cell cooperation). This effect

Table 4.4 Cells concerned with initiation of immune response

Cell	Essential functions
Macrophages	Remove and catabolize excess antigen. Localize and retain antigen at 'critical sites' and present antigen to lymphocytes. Regulate activities of lymphocytes by soluble factors. Bind antigen-antibody complexes by Fc and C3 receptors.
T lymphocytes	Act as 'helper' cells for certain antigens (T-dependent). Regulate activities of macrophages and B lymphocytes and recruit other T lymphocytes by soluble factors. 'Production of 'IgT' cytophilic for macrophages for presentation of antigen to B lymphocytes.
B lymphocytes	Immunoglobulin production. Binding of antigen by Ig receptors and responding to T-independent antigens. Fc and C3 receptors binding antigen-antibody complexes and possible role in activating the B lymphocytes and regulating their activity.

is called the **carrier effect** and was originally shown using haptenic groups such as dinitrophenol (DNP) attached to a protein carrier like bovine gamma globulin (BGG) or ovalbumin (OA). T cells appear to recognize the carrier and B cells the hapten. An animal immunized to DNP-BGG would not respond to a subsequent challenge with DNP-OA, indicating the need for T cells to recognize the carrier before B cells could respond to the hapten.

It seems probable that B cell activation and antibody synthesis can be the end result of a number of different stimuli, and that **macrophages, B cells** and **T cells** may all contribute in varying degrees, depending on the nature of the antigen, the dose of antigen and its mode of presentation.

The role of macrophages in antibody production
Macrophages play an important role in the **initiation of the immune response** by T and B lymphocytes. It has been known for some years that macrophages are required in order to obtain an immune response to sheep red blood cells by mouse spleen cells *in vitro*, and these findings have since been confirmed with a number of

antigens and in different species. The source of the macrophages was found to be important, and whilst those from the spleen or peritoneal cavity were effective, macrophages from the lung (alveolar macrophages) and liver (Kuppfer cells) were not able to co-operate with lymphocytes in the initiation of an immune response. The latter cells do, however, possess many features–functional and morphological–of macrophages, including the ability to adhere to glass, to phagocytic particles and to be cytotoxic for antibody coated cells.

Immune responses induced *in vitro* in spleen cell suspensions suggest that the macrophage appears to be necessary for an immune response to occur to T-dependent antigens (see above) and its presence has been shown to be necessary for the triggering of B lymphocytes by at least some T-independent antigens. Exactly how the macrophage helps in the processes leading to antibody production is not clear but the 'sticky' surface properties of the cell and its ability to take up antigen-antibody complexes and even T cell products, may enable the macrophage to present antigen to B cells in such a form as to trigger those cells for antibody production.

Macrophages may also function by **concentrating antigen** in 'critical sites', such as the follicles and medulla of the lymph nodes, thereby optimizing the chances of contact with lymphocytes. A further possibility is suggested by recent work indicating that macrophages can release 'soluble factors' (sometimes referred to as lymphocyte-activating factors–LAF) that can influence the activity of lymphocytes. The relative importance of these various macrophage activities in antibody production remains to be determined.

Some antigen may be retained at the surface of macrophages where it serves as a **depot of antigen** for the maintenace of the immune response. It is also possible that some antigen retained within the macrophage will function in this way although antigen can also be **catabolized** within the macrophage and later eliminated from the body as breakdown products. Macrophages have receptors for the Fc component of immunoglobulin and for C3b (p. 19). These will enable complexes of antibody and antigen to adhere to the macrophage membrane and be subsequently internalized.

Immune tolerance
Another possible result of the interaction of certain types of antigen, e.g. soluble protein antigens, with the surface of lymphocytes is that

the cell is prevented in some way from transforming for antibody production and is thus functionally eliminated from further participation in the immune response. This phenomenon is known as **immune tolerance** and is specific for the inducing antigen, and the term is used by immunologists to indicate a state in which the individual is unable to respond to a specific antigen or hapten. The phenomenon was recognized in 1924 by Glenny and Hopkins and also following the observation of Owen in 1945 that dizygotic cattle twins, parabiosed *in utero* by placental fusion, were permanent chimeras with respect to their red cells. Immune tolerance was first studied experimentally, by Medawar and his colleagues in mice injected neonatally with cells from another strain of mice (i.e. containing transplantation antigens) (p. 107). The injected mice were later able to accept grafts from the strain of mice which had donated the original injected cells. It has since been found that tolerance to a large variety of antigens can be readily induced when the antigens are injected neonatally. Tolerance can also be induced in the adult provided more antigen is given to take into account the maturity of the lymphoid system, the larger size of the lymphoid organs and thus the more cells to paralyse. A notable advance was made in this field when Mitchison using serum protein antigens showed that there was another form of tolerance inducible by very small doses of antigen. This was termed **low zone tolerance** in contrast to the high zone tolerance previously described. Doses between these two levels were found to immunize. Other workers have confirmed these findings with different types of antigen. Tolerance induced in either the T cell or B cell populations of lymphocytes results (as would be predicted from what is known of co-operation between the two cell populations) in tolerance of the whole animal to the antigen used to induce tolerance. This was established by transferring either tolerant T cells or tolerant B cells to a recipient mouse that had been irradiated and injected with normal cells of one or other population (i.e. T or B cells). Tolerant T cells would not co-operate with normal B cells to produce an immune response to human gammaglobulin and tolerant B cells would not co-operate with normal T cells to produce a response. The T cell population appeared to retain their tolerance for rather longer than the B cells (approximately 150 days compared to 50 days).

An additional complication has recently been noted by the finding that there appear to be two T cell populations. One cooperates with B cells to produce an immune response; the other appears to be able to inhibit or suppress B cells. **Suppressor T cells** seem to act early in the immune response and may be involved in the early stages of tolerance induction. They may act by recognizing the idiotypic determinants (p. 52) of the surface immunoglobulins of B cells and could be responsible for maintaining self-tolerance by suppressing those B cells expressing anti self immunoglobulin receptors.

Immunoglobulin synthesis

After the initial changes of transformation of lymphocytes have been set in motion, the actual **synthesis** of large amounts of immunoglobulin takes place. Two types of cell have been shown to be engaged in this process: (1) cells of the **plasmocytic** series and (2) cells of the **lymphocytic** series (small, medium and large lymphocytes). Of these two types the plasma cell line makes the largest contribution to immunoglobulin production and when single cells from immunized animals are examined in microdrops it can be shown that two-thirds of the **antibody producing cells** are of this type (Fig. 4.15). An important characteristic of any cell making immunoglobulin is the presence of a **rough endoplasmic reticulum** (formed by the attachment of protein-synthesizing polyribosomes to the convoluted endoplasmic reticulum membrane). The lymphocytes contain less of this than do plasma cells. It has been shown by a number of techniques that the immunoglobulin is localized in the spaces of the endoplasmic reticulum where it sometimes forms distinct aggregates termed Russell bodies.

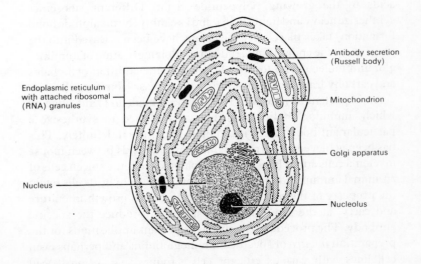

Fig. 4.15 Plasma cell.

In the spleen the cells engaged in antibody production tend to be found in the **red pulp**, and in the lymph glands in the **cortex**.

Individual immunoglobulin-producing cells appear to be able to synthesize the whole molecule, both heavy and light polypeptide chains (p. 50). It has also been found that the individual cells make only one class of immunoglobulin and that the light chains are restricted to only one of the two types (K and L, p. 50). It is very unusual to find an immunoglobulin secreting cell synthesizing more than one class of immunoglobulin although B cells in the early stages of an immune response can be shown to be secreting IgM antibody. They later switch to the synthesis of IgG antibody and thus at any one time produce only one class of immunoglobulin. Recent evidence indicates that the same cell can switch back to IgM production during a secondary response. The IgG that is produced is of the same specificity as the earlier IgM and almost certainly involves continued synthesis of the same light chain and the same variable region of the heavy chain; only the constant region is altered. The genetic mechanism may be a translocation event whereby the variable region gene becomes dissociated from the μ constant region gene and associates with the γ constant region gene. This IgM-IgG switch seems very likely to depend upon the influence of T cells on the B cell population.

The actual synthesis of immunoglobulin (after DNA has directed the synthesis of the appropriate mRNA) is carried out on the ribosomes of the producing cell, tRNAs sequentially adding amino acids to the growing polypeptide chain. Different ribosomes synthesize heavy and light chains, and assembly (by disulphide bond formation) takes place after the chains have been released into the cisternae of the endoplasmic reticulum. Polymerization of immunoglobulin molecules to form IgM involves the addition of J chains and carbohydrate groups just prior to its release from the cell.

An important advance has recently been made in Cambridge by which immunoglobulin-producing cells primed to synthesize a particular antibody can be maintained in culture indefinitely. This has been achieved by forming lymphocyte hybrids between mouse myeloma cells and B lymphocytes separated from the spleen cells of an animal immunized to a particular antigen. The hybrid cells retain the property of the myeloma cell of continuous growth in culture and carry, at the same time, the ability to produce the specific antibody. The procedure clearly has important implications for the preparation *in vitro* of specific immunoglobulins and perhaps even cell lines with various effector cell activities, e.g. using T cell lymphoma cells.

Gut-associated lymphoid tissue and antibody production

The thymus appears to control the cells of the cell-mediated immune system (p. 77) probably by providing facilities for the maturation of immature bone marrow cells. The cells of the immune system concerned with producing circulating antibodies reside mainly in the cortico-medullary junction and medullary cords of lymph nodes and the red pulp of the spleen.

The first evidence that B lymphocytes might be influenced by a non-thymic lymphoid organ came from phylogenetic studies in neonatal chickens which failed to develop normal immunological capacity after removal of the gut-associated lymphoid organ known as the **bursa of Fabricius**. Thymectomized chickens, as would be expected from the discussion above, fail to develop cell-mediated immune processes whilst capable of a humoral immune response. In striking contrast, bursectomized chicken fail to make immunoglobulins and have no plasma-cells or germinal centres in the lymphoid organs. Their cell-mediated mechanisms are, on the other hand, intact. Evidence is now emerging which suggests that there is a traffic of bursal lymphocytes to germinal centres in the spleen and lymph nodes comparable to that described in the thymus for bone marrow lymphocytes.

The search for an equivalent of the bursa in mammals, including man, is not yet complete but the evidence suggests that the fetal liver is the primary site of B cell development and that the bone marrow takes over later.

THE CELLULAR PROCESSES
INVOLVED IN ANTIBODY FORMATION

Learning and memory. The outstanding feature underlying these mechanisms is that the immune response is a **learning process** at the cellular level.

After initial contact with an antigen the cells of the immune system retain a memory which can be evoked on subsequent contact with the antigen, and furthermore, like other learning processes, the immune system becomes increasingly skilled with continued experience of a particular antigen. The antibody which is synthesized becomes increasingly more effective in binding with antigens, as those cells which are best able to produce a 'good fitting' (avid) antibody molecule are selected from the population of antibody-forming cells. At the same time increasing numbers of committed cells are added to the immune system on repeated contact with antigen and the magnitude of the response is increased

(p. 42). This increase in quantity and **avidity** of antibody can lead for example to increased efficiency in neutralizing an infective agent or its toxic products so that a well-immunized animal would be able to withstand a dose of the agent which might be lethal to a poorly immunized animal.

There is at present no satisfactory explanation of the cellular mechanisms which lead to the evocation of either the antibody response or the cell-mediated immune response. This state of affairs is not due to lack of speculation and experimentation, since in the last few years much effort has been directed at solving these problems.

Theories of antibody production
Two main theories have evolved which account for antibody synthesis and are referred to as **directive** and **selective** theories.

Directive theory. The **directive** theory was formulated by Haurowitz, Mudd and Alexander in the early 1930s and later modified by Pauling. The antigen is visualized as a mould or template which can enter any immunoglobulin producing cell and cause the pattern of amino acids laid down to be modified so that it will fit the template, resulting in the synthesis of a molecule with a spatial configuration complementary to that of the antigen molecule. To account for the continued production of antibody it is assumed that the antigen, or part of it, remains in the cell to direct future antibody production. Alternatively, it is proposed that the antigen modifies the genetic information in the DNA of the cell so that it and its daughter cells continue to produce the specific immunoglobulin.

Selective theory. In contrast, the **selective** theory proposes that antigen selects, from the population of cells capable of making antibody, only those few cells that already have the inherent ability to make an immunoglobulin specific for the antigen, the antigen serving simply as a trigger on reacting as suggested above with antibody receptor sites at the lymphocyte cell membrane. **The clonal selection theory** of Burnet is the best known of the selective theories and was formulated and modified over the years to take account of the hitherto unexplained phenomenon of recognition by the normal individual of tissue antigens as part of self and distinguishing these from foreign non-self antigens. Such an explanation became necessary with the description of human diseases where self recognition breaks down and self antigen is treated as if it were foreign antigen – resulting in so-called autoimmune disease (p. 142). The theory proposes that the cells of the antibody-forming system have arisen by random mutation resulting in the emergence of small numbers of cells or clones of cells differentiated so as to be capable of producing one or a very small number of specific antibodies. Contact by such differentiated cells during fetal life before the cells have reached maturity, with self or foreign antigenic material, would lead to suppression rather than stimulation of antibody formation against the particular antigen concerned – **immune tolerance**. That this could occur was illustrated by the experiments of Medawar and his colleagues on mice which could be induced to accept potentially incompatible skin grafts by pretreatment during neonatal life with the appropriate 'transplantation antigen'. These studies were the forerunner of much further work in this field and it has now been shown that tolerance can also be induced even in adult animals if antigen is given in suitable doses and in an appropriate manner. However, it is more difficult to do this in the adult, the immature immune system of the neonatal animal being more susceptible. X-irradiation of an adult is frequently used as an aid in tolerance induction (p. 64).

Burnet has since suggested that the initial contact with self antigens leading to the elimination of 'self-reactive clones' or 'forbidden clones', may take place in the thymus, this organ acting as a **censor** of the lymphoid cells. This idea is supported by the very rapid turnover of lymphocytes in that organ and by the emergence of self-reactive antibody-producing cells in the absence of the thymus. The view is held by some immunologists that the ageing process may in part be due to a failure in these proposed controlling mechanisms, i.e. a gradual loss of efficiency of the censorship role of the thymus associated with its atrophy later in life.

The immune response to an antigen and the consequences of repeated stimulation can readily be explained in terms of the selective theory.

Antigen introduced into an animal comes in contact with lymphocytes carrying receptors corresponding to the antigenic determinants of the antigen molecule (p. 23). Some receptors (high affinity receptors) will fit the determinant well whilst others (low affinity receptors) will not fit so well. The dose of antigen given will have an effect on whether more antigen is bound by high or low affinity receptors – the less antigen given, the greater the chance that cells with high affinity receptors will bind antigen. With increasing doses of antigen more will be available to combine with the lymphocytes with the weaker lower affinity receptors. The consequence of this is that large doses of antigen will generate antibody of low average affinity and small doses will generate high affinity antibody. On subsequent administration of antigen, antibodies of progressively **higher affinity** will be produced. This is because after the first dose of antigen its concentration will gradually fall in the tissues as it is gradually catabolized and eliminated, this will result in less antigen being available for the lymphocytes with low affinity receptors. In these circumstances as indicated above, lymphocytes with high affinity receptors will preferentially bind the small amounts of antigen remaining and will consequently be stimulated to produce high affinity antibody. This 'selection' of lymphocytes will be reflected in the **affinity** of the antibody stimulated by subsequent doses of antigen given to the immunized animal.

Implications and variations of theories. The theory outlined above suggests that early contact with self antigens leads to the individual developing an immune system which is suppressed or is tolerant towards self antigens. The unblocking of a cell inherently capable of producing antibody against self antigen would explain **auto-antibody** formation (p. 142). It is for this aspect of immunity in particular that the clonal selection theory provides a more plausible explanation than the directive theory which requires that all antibody-forming cells are blocked by every self antigen rather than only those cells capable of responding specifically to each antigen concerned. The other main characteristics of antibody formation – the specificity of antibody for antigen and the differences between the primary and secondary responses – can be explained equally well by either theory; the clonal selection theory is however the most complete attempt so far to take into account all the known facts of antibody production.

A number of variations of Burnet's original selective hypothesis have been proposed in the last few years but all maintain the assumption that the cell is already programmed to produce a specific antibody. It has been postulated, for example, that each potentially immunologically competent cell carries chromosomal DNA genes for a large variety of different types of antibody and is thus capable of responding to many antigens (sometimes referred to as the 'germ line theory'). An alternative proposal is that all antibody-producing cells may initially make identical immunoglobulins but during the lifetime of the individual variability of amino acid sequence appears due to crossing over during mitosis of the nucleotides responsible for coding the

variable amino acid sequences of the Fab portion of the molecule. There is a clear survival value in such a variation producing mechanism resulting in the production of immunoglobulins capable of reacting with a wide range of environmental antigens. Similarly there is survival value in the maintenance of those parts of the gene carrying the nucleotide sequences for the **constant** parts of the immunoglobulin molecule which maintain its structural integrity.

In conclusion immunologists have yet to resolve the question as to whether the wide range of antibody specificity found in the adult animal is the result of **somatic mutation** within the lymphocyte population or whether the necessary information is encoded in the inherited **germ line** cells. Recent work by Milstein and his colleagues at Cambridge, using cultures of clones of mouse myeloma cell lines, showed some cells producing immunoglobulin which varied from that produced by other cells of the same clone. This suggests that somatic mutation had occurred in the structural genes coding for immunoglobulin heavy chains. This evidence is further supported by workers in Australia who removed single antibody forming cells from a clone of cells and showed that in some cases their progeny were producing slightly different antibody. Evidence obtained by measuring the rate at which labelled messenger RNA or labelled DNA anneals with single stranded DNA from the parent genome indicates that there are probably only a small number of genes coding for the variable regions of the immunoglobulin molecule. This would argue strongly for somatic mutation as the **generator of antibody diversity**.

The idea that an antigen selects and reacts with a pre-existing lymphocyte receptor specific for the antigenic determinant should not be interpreted too strictly. It is inconceivable that each individual carries an infinite number of lymphocytes with appropriate receptors for an infinite number of antigenic determinants. Remembering that the combining site of an antibody molecule recognizes the shape of an antigenic determinant (p. 23) then one combining site will be able to recognize two or more antigenic determinants with very similar (although not identical) shapes (Fig. 4.16). It has been estimated that a minimum of 10^4–10^5 antibody combining sites (existing as receptors on lymphocytes) are required to provide the 'shapes' necessary to combine with all possible antigenic determinants.

THE CELL-MEDIATED ACQUIRED IMMUNE RESPONSE

In the immunologically mature individual, contact with an antigen

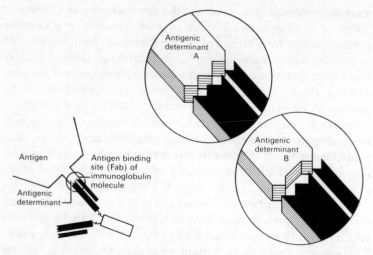

Fig. 4.16 Diagrammatic view of combining ability of an antibody molecule directed primarily at antigenic determinant A but able to combine also (cross react) with antigenic determinant B. The strength of the bond will be less when the antibody is combined with determinant B as the molecules will be in less close apposition (see p. 172).

leads not only to the production of circulating antibody, but also to the development of a separate cell-mediated form of response. In both types initial contact with the antigen is necessary and the response is specific for the antigen. Cell-mediated immunity occurs particularly in infections by agents which enter the cells such as viruses, tubercle bacilli and *Brucella* species (p. 123). It can also develop after skin contact with certain simple chemical substances (p. 104). The sequence of steps leading to this form of immunity is essentially no different from that leading to the antibody response but the response is initiated in different areas of the spleen and lymph nodes (white pulp around the central arterioles of the spleen and the paracortical areas of the lymph nodes); these areas are under the control of the thymus gland (p. 77). A characteristic of these thymus-dependent lymphocytes is that they can be stimulated to differentiate and divide by plant extracts known as phytohaemag-glutinins (PHA) and by certain extracts of microorganisms such as streptolysin S from streptococci. These substances, sometimes referred to as mitogens, appear to act on the small lymphocytes of all vertebrates so far examined and induce enlargement of the cells, increased synthesis of RNA followed later by DNA synthesis. The plant extracts are specific for sugar determinants present in the lymphocyte cell membrane, and interaction leads to 'triggering' of

Table 4.5 Main steps in lymphocyte transformation

1. Reaction of inducer at plasma membrane – PHA or antigen

2. Increased synthesis of RNA in 30 min to 2 hours

3. Morphological changes – enlargement of the cell, changes in nucleus,
   (transformation)   increases in lysosome granules and endocytosis
                              (commences at about 20 hours)

4. Increase in thymidine incorporation into DNA about 36 hours for
   PHA and 40 hours for antigens. Mitosis

the activity of the cell. This involves biochemical changes that are now beginning to be understood and include transport of ions (e.g. Ca^{++}), amino acids and nucleotides through the cell membrane leading to purine synthesis and finally cell division. This process is known as **lymphocyte transformation** and can be brought about in sensitized lymphocytes on subsequent exposure to the sensitizing antigen. (See Table 4.5.) Transformation is readily measured *in vitro* by culturing the cells in the presence of labelled precursors of nucleic acids, e.g. ^{14}C thymidine for DNA synthesis or ^{14}C uridine for RNA synthesis. The test can be used to detect sensitization to an antigen and the non-specific plant mitogens are used as a test of the competence of the cell-mediated immune system. Lymphocytes from an individual with, for example, an immune deficiency state (chap. 5) with thymic aplasia and consequent defective cell-mediated immunity would be unable to transform in the presence of PHA. Transformation of lymphocytes to PHA is reduced in certain virus infections (p. 129).

Mechanisms of cell-mediated immunity

Lymphocyte activation products
Cell-mediated immunity dependent on those activated lymphocytes is usually recognized by means of a skin test (e.g. intradermal injection) with the antigen that, in an individual who has developed a cell-mediated immune response, results in an inflammatory reaction at the injection site. When examined histologically it can be seen that the tissues at the injection site have been infiltrated by mononuclear cells, mainly lymphocytes and a few macrophages. There is considerable experimental evidence that the majority of the infiltrating cells are not the activated (or sensitized) lymphocytes that have previously been sensitized to antigen but uncommitted cells attracted by soluble products of the sensitized lymphocytes.

Lymphokines. There are soluble products of activated lymphocytes (sometimes called lymphocyte activation products – LAPs) produced by exposure of sensitized lymphocytes to the sensitizing antigen. They are believed to serve three main functions: (1) **recruitment** of uncommitted lymphocytes, (2) **retention** of such cells and phagocytes at the inflammatory site and (3) **activation** of the retained cells so that they can take part in the inflammatory response. These products can be thought of as chemical messengers that allow **communication** between the cells and also as agents that **amplify** the response. They act on macrophages, polymorphs, lymphocytes and also on other non-lymphoid cells.

The best known of these non-antibody factors released by sensitized lymphocytes on contact with antigen has the property of preventing the *in vitro* migration of macrophages on a glass surface. Macrophages can be set up in culture in small capillary tubes and will normally migrate out of the open end of the tube into the culture fluid (Fig. 4.17). A factor released from lymphocytes

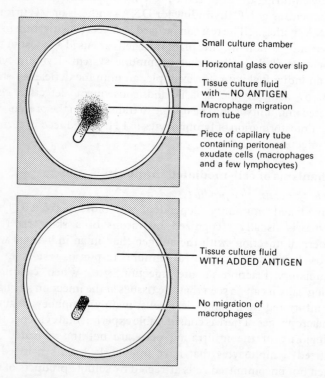

Small culture chamber

Horizontal glass cover slip

Tissue culture fluid with — NO ANTIGEN

Macrophage migration from tube

Piece of capillary tube containing peritoneal exudate cells (macrophages and a few lymphocytes)

Tissue culture fluid WITH ADDED ANTIGEN

No migration of macrophages

Fig. 4.17 Macrophage migration inhibition test

exposed to antigen will prevent this migration by causing the macrophages to stick together. This factor is likely to be released also *in vivo* and may be responsible for the accumulation of macrophages in cell-mediated immune reactions (p. 73). Purification and identification of those factors are very different as they are produced in very small amounts. Guinea pig macrophage inhibitory factor appears to be a glycoprotein with a molecular weight of 35–50,000, but its mechanism of action is unknown. Another probably different factor that affects macrophages has the property of activating the cells. Such activated macrophages can be shown to have increased bacteriocidal activity as well as activity against tumour cells (p. 170). A further as yet undefined factor released from sensitized lymphocytes after exposure to antigen causes stimulation and proliferation of normal unsensitized lymphocytes. This is known as mitogenic factor. Yet another lymphokine has a chemotactic effect on macrophages attracting them to the site of the inflammatory response. A cytotoxic effect, which appears to be due to a lymphokine (lymphotoxin), has also been demonstrated with a damaging effect on a variety of types of cell. A factor which increases capillary permeability (skin reactive factor) can also be shown to be released by sensitized lymphocytes. A number of as yet uncharacterized factors have been described that appear to modulate antibody production by B cells. Some are able to enhance B cell activity whilst others suppress antibody production.

The overall contribution of these factors in the cell-mediated immune response has not yet been clearly established nor has their chemical identity or mode of action. However, it is widely believed that the lymphokines are the main effector mechanisms in the cell-mediated responses. When *in vitro* prepared lymphokines are injected into guinea-pig lymph nodes, lymphocytes accumulate in the paracortical region and there is enlargement of follicles with mitotic activation in germinal centres. A possible adjuvant effect is suggested for lymphokines as lymph node injection leads to an enhanced response to injected antigen. Lymphokines can be recovered in the afferent lymph in the primary immune response in a lymph node and can be recovered from explants of granulomata in culture (e.g. schistosomia granulomata, p. 133), and in rheumatoid synovial fluids. Intradermal injection of lymphokines induces exudation of plasma proteins and inflammatory cells, and intraperitoneal injection aggregates macrophages in the intraperitoneal fluid exudate. Table 4.6 shows some of these lymphocyte activation products and the suggested *in vivo* activities of the factors.

Table 4.6

Lymphokine activity	Possible role *in vivo*
Macrophage 'migration inhibition'	Retention of emigrated macrophages at site of inflammation
Macrophage 'chemotaxis'	Emigration of macrophages to site of inflammation
Macrophage 'activation'	Enhanced metabolic, phagocytic and anti-microbial activities
Macrophage 'aggregation'	Aggregation and localization of macrophages at inflammatory site.
Macrophage 'arming'	Enhanced extracellular cytotoxic effects of macrophages
Macrophage 'spreading-inhibition'	Brings about cell surface changes possibly facilitating passage of cells through blood vessel walls
Lymphocyte 'mitogenesis'	Induces non-committed lymphocytes to become metabolically active at inflammatory site
Lymphocyte 'potentiation'	Augmentation of lymphocyte activation by specific antigen
Lymphocyte 'suppression'	Limitation of DNA synthesis by lymphocytes
Lymphocyte 'co-operation'	Facilitation of B cell response to T-dependent antigens.
Granulocyte 'migration inhibition'	Similar effect as on macrophages
Granulocyte 'chemotaxis inhibition'	Similar effect as on macrophages
'Cytotoxic' effects	Induces lymphocyte cytotoxicity on certain cell types
'Inhibition of proliferation'	Inhibition of cell proliferation without lysis
'Virus suppression'	Interferon-like factors protecting from virus infection

In vivo *role of cell-mediated immunity*

It seems likely that the cell-mediated immune response is involved in protection against various infective agents (p. 127). It may also serve an important physiological role in the normal individual bringing about the elimination of spontaneously arising neoplastic cells which might represent a potential threat to the individual. In support of the existence of such an **immunological surveillance** mechanism (chap. 11) it has been found that the incidence of tumours is highest at the two extremes of life when the immunological mechanisms are at their least efficient. The cell-mediated immune system is under the influence of the thymus and the cells are referred to as thymus dependent or T cells, after thymectomy in mice the incidence of tumours induced by chemical carcinogens and viruses has been found to be significantly higher than in sham-thymectomized controls. The thymus has been found to be absent in certain rare immune deficiency states of children (p. 90). In such conditions there is a deficiency of lymphocytes from the areas of spleen and lymph nodes under thymic control. Cell-mediated immune reactions are absent and there is an inability to deal with virus infections. This type of cell-mediated immune mechanism would be likely to have arisen **early in evolution** with the development of multicellular organisms and would have additional survival value in that it would also be effective against exogenous parasites.

The role of the thymus in immune reactivity

Development and structure. The thymus in mammals arises from the endoderm of the third and fourth branchial clefts and is the tissue in which lymphocytes can first be recognized. The thymus gland increases in size until puberty and then slowly atrophies although it is still readily recognizable in the adult. The cells of the thymus are of three main types: **thymocytes** morphologically similar to blood lymphocytes, **phagocytic reticulum cells** and **reticular epithelial cells.** The macroscopic structure of the organ is like that of other lymphoid organs in general organization, with a central medulla containing a high proportion of reticular cells and a peripheral cortex containing the thymocytes with some surrounding reticular cells. Unlike the spleen and lymph nodes there are no germinal centres and no plasma cells. Thus under normal physiological conditions the thymus cells do not make antibody. Plasma cells will appear only if antigen is injected directly into the organ. Hassall's corpuscles are a feature peculiar to the medulla of the thymus and consist of groups of reticular epithelial cells sometimes flattened and concentrically arranged around a central core of nuclear debris.

Cell turnover and humoral factors. The thymus can be shown, by tritiated thymidine incorporation studies, to be actively engaged in lymphopoiesis, there being a higher proportion of primitive actively dividing lymphoid cells than in any other lymphoid tissue such as the spleen or lymph nodes, and with a correspondingly high mitotic rate. Evidence suggests that the stimulus for thymocytes to divide arises in some way from the reticular epithelial cells. The primitive cells in the thymus are slowly replaced during life by cells derived from the bone marrow that migrate via the blood stream into the thymus. A small proportion of these cells leave the thymus and find their way to the peripheral lymphoid tissues; these are the **long-lived lymphocytes** with a life of months in rodents and possibly years in man.

Maturation of T cells during the period they spend in the thymus has been shown to take place. The changes associated with this can be detected by means of **membrane antigens** on the T lymphocytes. The main murine antigen markers are known as Thy (theta), TL and Ly antigens. The TL antigen is present on the lymphocytes that enter the thymus but is lost on maturation in the gland. The amount of Thy antigen is also much reduced during this period and the Ly antigens develop and are expressed on mature T lymphocytes. Various functional characteristics have been found to be associated with different Ly antigens and T lymphocytes carrying such antigens can thus be divided into **subpopulations**. The functional activities that can be defined on the basis of Ly markers are 'helper cell activity' (see cell cooperation, p. 79), cytolysis of allogeneic lymphocytes or tumour cells, i.e. 'cytotoxic T cells' and 'suppressor cell' activity involved in controlling B lymphocytes (see p. 64).

If the thymus is removed during the neonatal period, it is possible to find lymphocyte-deficient areas in the white pulp of the spleen around the central arterioles and in the paracortical area of the lymph nodes. These areas have been termed the '**thymus-dependent**' areas of the lymphoid tissues. Associated with this localized deficiency of lymphocytes, neonatally thymectomized animals also have considerably impaired cell-mediated immune effector mechanisms affecting graft rejection and other forms of cell-mediated immunity such as delayed hypersensitivity reactions; humoral immune reactivity is much less markedly affected.

Studies in mice of cell turnover in the adult thymus show that the thymic population of lymphocytes is replaced every three or four days but that the great majority of cells never leave the organ and die there. The reasons for this **intense lymphopoiesis** is unknown. In the adult it seems that the thymus is necessary for repopulation of lymphoid tissues depleted by X-irradiation or other methods. However, studies with chromosome markers have shown that the new cells are not derived directly from the thymus but are lymphoid cells from elsewhere in the body, probably from the bone marrow. The role of the thymus in this situation appears to be the production not of thymus-derived cells but of a humoral factor, **thymosin**, which restores immunological reactivity to remaining lymphoid cells. This was strongly suggested by experiments in which thymus implants in millipore diffusion chambers were placed in the peritoneal cavity of thymectomized mice. Immunological capacity was restored to the recipients, which recovered the ability to reject skin grafts, although the chambers were impermeable to cells and were on later recovery shown to contain only reticular epithelial and reticulum cells and no lymphocytes.

The essential functions of the thymus can be summarized as bringing about the **differentiation** and **proliferation** of primitive bone marrow-derived lymphoid cells and producing a **humoral factor** with the ability to induce immunological competence in lymphocytes. Immunologists are unfortunately as yet some way from understanding fully the exact mechanisms of interaction between the gland and the peripheral lymphoid tissues.

It is worth noting at this point that the hormonal factor produced by the thymus is not the only hormonal influence acting on the lymphoid tissues. **Growth hormone** increases thymus weight and thyroid hormone increases the weight of the lymphoid tissues and the size of the immune response. Adrenalectomy also increases the weight of the lymphoid tissues, and **glucocorticoids, oestrogens** and **androgens** decrease its weight. After neonatal thymectomy acidophilic growth hormone producing cells of the anterior pituitary appear to lose their granules suggesting an increased demand for output of hormone by the cells in the absence of the thymus. Interference with the production of **anterior pituitary** hormones in mice by means of specific antisera results in lymphocyte depletion in both thymus and spleen. All these observations indicate the close relationship between endocrinological function, immunological maturation and expression of immune capacity.

CELL COOPERATION

Central and peripheral lymphoid tissues

Knowledge of immune-reactivity which is either thymus-dependent or bursa-dependent has led to the concept of separate **central** and **peripheral** lymphoid tissues. The central organs—the thymus and the bursa of Fabricius (or its equivalent in mammals, initially fetal liver and later bone marrow)—are responsible for development and control of the peripheral lymphoid tissues—the spleen and lymph nodes.

A tentative scheme showing the possible inter-relationships of central and peripheral lymphoid tissues is given in Figure 4.18. Experimental work, based on repopulation of irradiated animals by

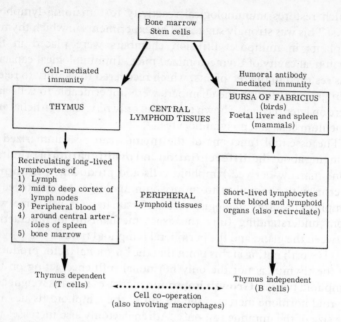

Fig. 4.18 Scheme illustrating possible relationship between central and peripheral lymphoid tissues.

lymphoid cells from different origins, indicates that for the expression of at least some forms of immune response, there is co-operation between cells in the peripheral lymphoid tissues derived directly from the bone marrow and lymphocytes derived from the thymus. The former cells are referred to as **B cells** (bone marrow derived) and the latter as **T cells** (thymus-dependent). The B cells are responsible for **immunoglobulin synthesis** and may sometimes be directly stimulated by contact with antigen–usually powerful antigens such as salmonella flagellin or haemocyanin. Other weaker antigens such as serum albumin require the co-operation of T cells acting as **helper cells** leading in some way to an immune response by the B cells. T cells and macrophages may, for example, concentrate antigen and present it to B cells; or perhaps T cells may release soluble factors (p. 61) to stimulate B cells (see p. 60 and Section on cell co-operation and genetic control p. 84). T and B cells are morphologically indistinguishable until they transform after antigenic stimulation. The cytoplasm of transformed T lymphocytes can be seen under the electron microscope to contain numerous polyribosomes, in contrast the transformed B cell is packed with rough endoplasmic reticulum followed by the appearance of intra cytoplasmic vesicles of antibody (p. 65, Fig. 4.15). Both T and B cell populations show a similar change in their behaviour after primary and secondary antigenic stimulation the cell populations both increase in size and develop immunological memory. Initially the B cells produce IgM antibody and then switch to IgG production coincident with this change the surface receptors on these B cells change from IgM to IgG type (see p. 66).

T lymphocyte receptors
There is much discussion among immunologists about the nature of the receptor for antigen on T lymphocytes. Immunoglobulins that resemble the monomeric subunits of IgM have been isolated from T lymphocytes. Their detection depends upon incorporating a radioactive label into the membrane immunoglobulin. Released labelled immunoglobulin can then be detected in the culture medium of the T lymphocyte preparations. The immunoglobulin detected in this way appears to have a particular ability to attach to cells thought to be macrophages. It is suggested that this T cell immunoglobulin assists in the initiation of the immune response by trapping antigen on the macrophage surface, where it is presented to B cells that are then triggered to produce antibody. Not all immunologists are convinced that the 'T cell immunoglobulin' (sometimes called IgT) is actually produced by the T cell but that it may be taken up passively after being produced by B lymphocytes. However, certain T cell lines kept in culture are claimed to actively synthesize a T cell immunoglobulin, but it remains to be established if this is an *in vitro* artefact not reflected in normal T lymphocyte populations *in vivo*. Other T cell products of non-immunoglobulin nature have been described which appear to assist B cells to respond to antigen and this is discussed on p. 75.

Recent work on the **genetic control** of the immune response (see p. 84) has led to the suggestion that the antigen binding site on T cells is closely linked to (or even part of) a product of the gene complex controlling the histocompatibility antigens of the cell membrane and coded for by the **immune response (Ir) genes** of this complex (see p. 84). The precise nature of the T cell receptor is, however, still highly controversial, and other investigators using specific antisera claim that B cells and macrophages, rather than T cells, express the antigens coded for by the Ir genes. This means that the Ir gene products may not themselves be the receptor for antigen, but in the T cell they may perhaps control the functioning of a specific antigen receptor on the T cell.

Cellular traffic in other lymphoid tissues

In a previous section (p. 78) consideration was given to the traffic of lymphocytes from the bone marrow via the thymus to the lymph nodes. This journey, during which the cells are maturing and proliferating, probably takes a period of weeks. Another form of lymphocytic traffic also exists involving a non-dividing population of small lymphocytes with a potential life span of many months and derived mainly from the thymus. This journey is measured in hours rather than days (Fig. 4.19). This traffic takes the form of a **recirculation** of small lymphocytes between the blood and lymphoid tissue, and thus each small lymphocyte may be exchanged between these two compartments very many times during its lifetime. One of the main advantages to the individual of such a recirculation process is that, for example, during the course of a natural infection the continual traffic of lymphocytes would enable very many different lymphocytes to have **access to the antigen** with the result that there would be a good chance that a lymphocyte carrying antibody receptor for the particular antigen would come across it and initiate an immune reaction. Another possible role of this recirculation process is that it can be used to **replenish** the

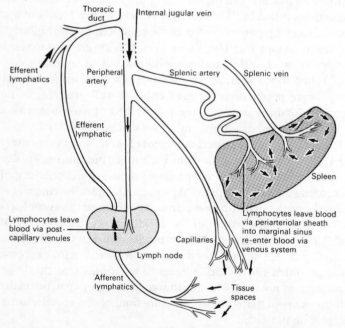

Fig. 4.19 Schematic view of main pathways of lymphocyte circulation.

lymphoid tissue of, for example, the spleen which might have been depleted by X-irradiation, trauma or infection.

There is convincing evidence that lymphoid tissues can **recruit** lymphocytes from the recirculating pool. If a rat spleen is irradiated immediately after an intravenous injection of sheep red cells the antibody response is only slightly delayed. However, if whole body irradiation is given after the initial splenic irradiation there is complete suppression of the anti-sheep cell response. It thus seems likely that without whole body irradiation the irradiated spleen is able to recruit a fresh supply of lymphocytes from the circulating pool.

Another situation in which recirculation of lymphocytes could be helpful in the induction of an immune response is where the local concentration of antigen might be sufficient to induce tolerance rather than immunity in a static cell population. The passage of lymphocytes through an area where antigen had been localized and concentrated on the dendritic processes of macrophages might facilitate the induction of immunity.

The routes of lymphocyte recirculation

There are three main areas where the migration or transfer of lymphocytes from the blood takes place: the **lymph nodes** and Peyer's patches, the **spleen** and the peripheral **blood vessels**. Most is known about the mechanism of transfer in the lymph nodes where studies using the electron microscope show that small lymphocytes actually penetrate and traverse the cytoplasm of the cuboidal endothelial cells of the post-capillary venules. These **post-capillary venules** are confined to the deep and mid zones of the lymph node cortex and are unusual in that their endothelial cells are hypertrophied and cuboidal in appearance in comparison with the flattened endothelium of normal post-capillary venules found elsewhere. From the lymph node cortex the lymphocytes pass through the node to the medullary sinuses and then to the efferent lymphatics.

The precise routes of lymphocyte migration in the peripheral blood circulation are not clear, but the migration seems to be on a much smaller scale than in lymphoid tissues and almost certainly takes place across capillary walls. The flow can be increased if a local granuloma is formed in response to some foreign agent; then the migration from blood to lymph can be as great as in the lymph nodes themselves.

In the spleen, post-capillary venules have not been described and it appears that small lymphocytes enter the periarteriolar sheath from the blood, passing between the cells rather than through them as in the post-capillary venules. The cells later re-enter the blood within the spleen rather than leave via the lymphatics.

Cell co-operation and the genetic control of the immune response

Despite the wealth of experimental data, the conclusions of which have been summarized in the preceding paragraphs the precise mechanisms by which immunocompetent cells co-operate together to produce an immune response remains clouded in mystery. In the last few years new light, but by no means complete illumination, has been shed on the problem by the realization that certain genes controlling the ability of the immunocompetent cells to respond to antigen are genetically very closely related to those genes controlling certain important cell surface antigens. These antigens are those involved in rejection of grafts and on transfer of a graft of tissue to an unrelated (allogeneic) recipient are recognized as foreign. An immune response is initiated and the graft is rejected (see p. 109).

The cell surface antigens are known as **histocompatibility** antigens and the group of genes that determines the expression of these antigens as the **major histocompatibility complex** (MHC). In the mouse these genes are present in chromosome number 17 and, as has been noted above, are closely related in this chromosome to the genes that control the immune response– referred to as the immune response (**Ir**) **genes or I region**.

The I region appears to determine certain surface antigens on T and B lymphocytes. Some of these antigens can be found on both T and B cells whilst others appear to be restricted to one cell type. T helper cells (see p. 60) and B cells appear to both carry one of these antigens, whilst suppressor T cells (p. 64), only, carry another antigen. These I region determined surface antigens like the Ly antigens (p. 78) are likely to prove useful in subdividing lymphocyte cell populations with respect to their different functional activities.

The first clues that the MHC genes were involved in cell co-operation came from studies on collaboration between thymocytes and bone marrow cells in the immune response to sheep red blood cells. It was found that allogeneic thymocytes and bone marrow cells collaborate poorly and that the most efficient response was produced when the cells were from syngeneic donors. Genetic analysis revealed that concordance in the I region of the mouse MHC genes was necessary for efficient collaboration. The same conclusions have more recently been drawn from studies of collaboration between macrophages and lymphocytes.

The precise mechanisms underlying these effects are not clear but it is known that activation of T lymphocytes by antigen can be prevented by antisera directed against cell surface antigens controlled by the MHC genes. This suggested that the antisera were in some way blocking the receptor for antigen on T cells. Further studies have extended those observations and indicate that some gene product coded for by the MHC genes is involved in the steps that lead up to co-operation between T and B cells and possibly also in macrophage–T lymphocyte interactions. The nature of this gene product is not yet established, but recent work has indicated that in certain experimental systems in the mouse, a factor can be recovered from T lymphocytes that have been exposed to antigen (so-called educated T cells). This 'factor' can aid B lymphocytes in responses to certain antigens, and it seems possible that the factor may be the gene product involved in cell co-operation. The factor has been shown not to be an immunoglobulin and significantly is removed by antisera directed at MHC products. Immunologists await with interest identification of its chemical nature and the mechanism of its action on B lymphocytes.

The immunocyte complex

In this chapter the details have been set out of the origin of the immunoglobulins from lymphoid tissues and cells. The role of the thymus in influencing these cells has been described and an outline has been given of the traffic of lymphocytes between the various lymphoid organs. Details of the individual behaviour of particular cell population or tissues should not obscure the fact that the immune response is a highly complex process involving finely balanced **inter-relationships** between many different types of differentiated cell, e.g. macrophages, T lymphocytes, B lymphocytes, and influenced overall by the behaviour of the central lymphoid organs, e.g. the thymus and possibly other glandular tissues such as the pituitary.

The differentiated lymphoid cells involved in the immune response are all derived initially from the haemopoietic **stem cells** of the bone marrow. Bone marrow stem cells also differentiate to produce erythrocytes, thrombocytes, granulocytes and monocytes. The macrophages of the tissues and blood are derived from the latter cell. Figure 4.20 illustrates this schematically and shows the cells that make up what is referred to as the 'immunocyte complex' consisting of T and B lymphocytes capable of responding to antigen and called

antigen sensitive cells (or sometimes antigen reactive cells) and the cells which actually mediate the immune response and are actively committed to this; these cells are referred to as **immunocytes**.

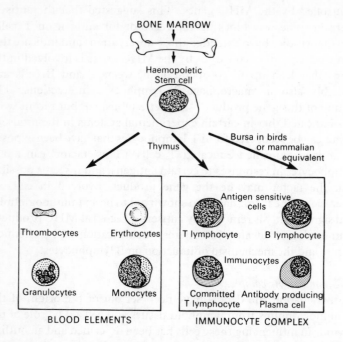

Fig. 4.20 Differentation of bone marrow derived stem cells into blood elements and the immunocyte complex.

FURTHER READING

Barrett, J. T. (1974) *Textbook of Immunology*. 2nd edition. London: Kimpton.

Bloom, B. R. (1971) *In vitro* approaches to the mechanism of cell-mediated immune reactions. *Adv. Immunol.*, **13,** 102.

Burnet, Sir Macfarlane. (1969) *Cellular Immunity*. Cambridge University Press.

Cohen, S., Humphrey, J. H. & Coombs, R. R. A. (1967) Antibodies structure and biological function. *Proc. R. Soc. Med.*, **60,** 589.

Cohen, S. & Milstein, C. (1967) Structure and biological properties of immunoglobulins. *Adv. Immun.*, **7,** 1.

Dresser, D. W. & Mitchison, N. A. (1968) The mechanism of immunological paralysis. *Adv. Immun.*, **8,** 129.

Edelman, G. M. (1970) The structure and function of antibodies. *Scient. Am.*, **223,** 34.

Ford, W. L. & Gowans, J. L. (1969) The traffic of lymphocytes. *Semin. Hemat.*, **6,** 67.

Marchalonis, J. J. (1976) *Comparative Immunology*. Oxford: Blackwell.

Hobart, M. J. & McConnell (1975) *The Immune System*. Oxford: Blackwell.

Hobbs, J. R. (1970) Immune globulins in some diseases. *Br. J. hosp. Med.*, **3**, 669.

Hudson, L. (1972) The cellular basis of the immune response. *Brit. J' hosp. Med.*, **8**, 648.

Humphrey, J. H. (1969) The fate of antigen and its relationship to the immune response. In *The Immune Response and its Suppression*, ed. Sorkin, E. Basel: Karger.

Humphrey, J. H. & White, R. G. (1970) *Immunology for Students of Medicine*. 3rd edition. Oxford: Blackwell.

Kabat, E. A. (1968) *Structural Concepts in Immunology and Immunochemistry*. New York: Holt, Rinehart & Winston.

Fudenberg, H. H., Stites, D. P., Caldwell, J. L. & Wells, J. V. (1976) *Basic and Clinical Immunology*. Los Altos: Lange.

Mitchison, N. A. (1968) Immunological paralysis as a dosage phenomenon. In *Regulation of the Antibody Response*, p. 54, ed. Cinader, B. Springfield, Illinois: Thomas.

Mitchison, N. A. (1972) Dose frequency and route of administration of antigen. In *Immunogenicity*, p. 87, ed. Borek, F. Amsterdam: North Holland.

Nelson, D. S. (Ed.) (1976) *Immunobiology of the Macrophage*. New York: Academic Press.

Nossal, G. J. V. (1967) Mechanisms of antibody production. *A. Rev. Med.*, **18**, 81.

Osaba, D. (1968) The regulatory role of the thymus in immunogenesis. In *Regulation of the Antibody Response*, p. 232, ed. Cinader, B. Springfield, Illinois: Thomas.

Pick, E. & Turk, J. L. (1972) The biological activities of soluble lymphocyte products. *Clin. exp. Immunol.*, **10**, 1.

Playfair, J. H. L. (1971) Cell cooperation in the immune response. *Clin. exp. Immun.*, **8**, 839.

Rogers Brambell, F. W. (1970) *The Transmission of Passive Immunity from Mother to Young*. Amsterdam: North Holland.

Rosenthal, A. S. (1975) *Immune Recognition*. New York: Academic Press.

Warner, N. L. (1972) Differentiation of immunocytes and evolution of immunological potential. In *Immunogenicity*, p. 467, ed. Borek, F. Amsterdam: North Holland.

Weiss, L. (1972) *The Cells and Tissues of the Immune System*. Englewood Cliffs, N.J.: Prentice-Hall.

White, R. G. (1967) Antigen adjuvants. In *Modern Trends in Immunology*, 2, p. 28, ed. Cruickshank, R. & Weir, D. M. London: Butterworth.

Wolstenholme, G. E. W. & Knight, J. (1970) *Hormones and the Immune Response*. Ciba Foundation Study Group No. 36. London: Churchill.

World Health Organization (1976) Immunological adjuvants. *Wld. Hlth. Org.*, Technical report series no. 595.

5

Defects in immunoglobulin synthesis and cell-mediated immune reactivity

The immunologically competent cells of the lymphoid tissues derived from, renewed and influenced by the activity of the thymus, bone marrow and probably gut associated lymphoid tissues, can be the subject of disease processes due either to defects in one of the components of the complex itself or secondarily to some other disease process affecting the normal functioning of some part of the lymphoid tissues. In 1953 Bruton first described hypo-gammaglobulinaemia in an 8-year-old boy who developed septic arthritis of the knee at 4 years of age followed by numerous attacks of otitis media, pneumococcal sepsis and pneumonia. Electrophoretic analysis of the serum proteins showed almost complete absence of the gamma-globulin fraction. The child appeared unable to give an immune response to typhoid and diphtheria immunization. It is now recognized that this form of deficiency is only one of a group of specific deficiencies affecting the lymphoid tissues which can affect both sexes, manifest themselves at any age and be genetically determined or arise secondarily to some other condition.

Primary defects

In the first category are the congenital defects affecting immuno-globulin synthetic mechanisms, cell-mediated immune mechanisms or sometimes both. Deficiency of immunoglobulin synthesis is complete in Bruton type agammaglobulinaemia an X-linked recessive character found in boys and in which the IgG level is reduced by about a tenth and the IgA and IgM about a hundredth of normal values. Cell-mediated immune mechanisms function normally in these patients who can reject grafts and develop normal delayed hypersensitivity to tuberculosis. However, they do not give the normal circulating antibody response to bacterial vaccines and are thus very susceptible to pyogenic infections. The lymphoid tissue in the appendix and Peyer's patches is somewhat reduced, and patients do not develop plasma cells and germinal centres in lymph nodes.

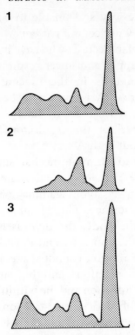

Fig. 5.1 Tracings obtained by ultraviolet scanning of electrophoretic patterns of human sera. (1) Normal Serum (2) Reduced gamma globulin (antibody deficiency syndrome possible B cell defect) (3) raised gamma globulin (possible myeloma). Peaks right to left: albumin, alpha, beta and gamma globulins (see Fig. 4.9).

Partial defects in immunoglobulin synthesis have been described affecting one or more of the main immunoglobulin classes. For example (a) the IgG or IgA levels may be reduced and the IgM level raised; (b) the IgA and IgM may be reduced and the IgG level be normal or (c) the IgA level may be reduced and the others normal.

Electrophoresis of serum as shown in Figure 5.1 cannot distinguish between the various immunoglobulin deficiencies and will only show gross changes in total immunoglobulins. Gel diffusion and immunoelectrophoretic techniques (p. 177) using anti-immunoglobulin antisera are required for the detailed analysis of these deficiencies.

In (a), which is inherited as an X-linked recessive character, the lymphoid tissues appear normal histologically although the plasma cells appear to be making predominantly IgM. Patients are susceptible to pyogenic infections and the condition is often associated with anaemia, thrombocytopoenia and neutropoenia. In (b) even the IgG which is produced in normal quantity is thought to be abnormal in some way and unable to combine with antigen. Defect (c) occurs in 80 per cent of patients with a condition known as hereditary ataxia telangiectasia who have increased susceptibility to infections of the upper and lower respiratory tract. There is a deficiency in plasma cells in the mucous membranes of the intestinal tract, where IgA is known to be produced in normal individuals, and the disease seems likely to be due to lack of protection at the level of the respiratory mucous membranes normally brought about by IgA secretion.

Both **cell-mediated** immune mechanisms and **immunoglobulin synthesis** are deficient in an X-linked disease of male children known as 'Swiss type agammaglobulinaemia' or severe combined immunodeficiency. There is almost complete absence of lymphoid tissue in the body, the thymus is very small and the lymphoid tissues of the appendix and Peyer's patches are absent. Children with this condition cannot make antibodies or develop cell-mediated immune reactions, and they suffer from progressive bacterial and/or viral infection and die within two years of birth.

In another type of deficiency state only the cell-mediated immune mechanisms are affected and there is thymic dysplasia and deficiency of lymphoid cells from those areas of the spleen and lymph nodes which are under thymic control. Although children with this rare type of deficiency can produce circulating antibody with their inability to develop cell-mediated immunity renders them highly susceptible to virus infection. One form of this condition associated with thymic dysplasia and absence of parathyroid glands is known as Di George's syndrome.

Secondary defects

Acquired deficiencies of the immunological mechanisms can occur secondarily to a number of disease states affecting the lymphoid tissues such as Hodgkin's disease, multiple myeloma, leukaemia and lymphosarcoma. Deficiency of immunoglobulins can also be brought about by excessive loss of protein through diseased kidneys or via the intestines in protein-losing enteropathy.

In contrast to the deficiency states just described, raised immunoglobulin levels are found in certain disorders of plasma cell function, which amount to malignant proliferation of a particular clone or family of plasma cells. In this condition known as multiple myeloma, a malignant clone is found to produce one particular class of immunoglobulin usually IgG or more rarely one of the other classes. The frequency of occurrence among myeloma of particular immunoglobulin classes reflects their relative levels in serum. There is usually a decreased synthesis of normal immunoglobulins associated with a deficient immune response to infective agents. On electrophoresis of serum a distinct band can be seen in the immunoglobulin area, and Figure 5.1 shows an example of the type of pattern found on simple paper electrophoresis. This abnormal band is produced by the raised levels of the myeloma immunoglobulin which is termed an M-type protein. In about 20 to 30 per cent of patients with multiple myeloma immunoglobulin light chains are found in the urine. These occur as dimers and are known as Bence-Jones protein. The condition is also associated with excess numbers of plasma cells in the bone marrow and X-ray evidence of myeloma cell deposits in bone.

Clinical aspects

Increased susceptibility to many types of infection is the outstanding feature of the immunological deficiency states. The age of onset of the congenital types is rarely earlier than 3 to 4 months of age due to the protective effects of maternal antibody. The most frequently affected site is the respiratory tract which is attacked by pyogenic bacteria or fungi. Lack of IgA antibody leads to particular susceptibility to chronic infection of the respiratory tract. Other clinical features frequently associated with immune deficiency states are skin rashes, diarrhoea, growth failure, enlarged liver and spleen and recurrent abscesses or osteomyelitis.

When there is deficiency of the cell-mediated immune mechanisms resistance to virus infections is diminished which may be recognized by the severe necrosis that will occur at the site of smallpox vaccination. BCG vaccination can lead to generalized tuberculosis infection in such cases.

Investigation of suspected immunological deficiency states should include family studies for any abnormalities of immune function. Lymphocyte function may be assessed by stimulation (a) with non-specific agents such as PHA or concanavalin A (p. 197) or (b) with a specific bacterial antigen in subjects previously sensitized to the bacterial antigen by natural infection or immunization (e.g. the tubercle bacillus). Quantitative determination of immunoglobulin levels can be made (p. 179) and estimation of the response to immunization with standard antigens. Peripheral blood counts and X-rays of the thymus region may also prove useful.

Treatment of deficiency states includes use of an appropriate antibiotic and regular administration of pooled human immunoglobulins. Closely matched sibling bone marrow has been used successfully in some cases and a graft of fetal thymus has been used

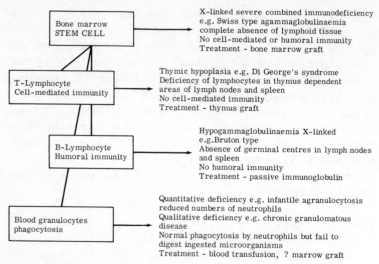

Fig. 5.2 Primary immunodeficiency and the cells of the immune system.

in the case of thymic aplasia. Figure 5.2 shows the components of the immune system with examples of deficiencies affecting them indicating the effects and possible forms of treatment.

Defective phagocytic mechanisms

These defects take two forms. (1) Where there is a **quantitative** deficiency of blood leucocytes which may be **congenital** (e.g. infantile agranulocytosis) or **acquired** as a result of replacement of bone marrow by tumour tissue or the toxic effects of chemicals. (2) Where there is a **qualitative** deficiency in the functioning of neutrophil leucocytes which whilst ingesting bacteria normally fail, because of an enzymic defect, to digest them. The clinical form of this defect is known as chronic granulomatous disease and is a sex-linked recessive condition characterized by increased susceptibility to infection in early life by microorganisms of low virulence to the normal individual.

FURTHER READING

Ammann, A. J. & Fudenberg, H. H. (1976) In *Basic and Clinical Immunology*, ed. Fudenberg, H. H., Stites, D. P., Caldwell, J. L. & Wells, J. V. Los Altos: Lange.

Asherson, G. L. (1972) The development of lymphocyte function tests. *Brit. J. hosp. Med.*, **8**, 665.

Gell, P. G. H., Coombs, R. R. A. & Lachmann, P. J. (1975) *Clinical Aspects of Immunology*. 3rd edition. Oxford: Blackwell.

Martin, N. H. (1970) The paraproteinaemias. *Br. J. hosp. Med.*, **3**, 662.

Turk, J. L. (1969) *Immunology in Clinical Medicine*. London: Heinemann.

Waldenstrom, J. G. (1968) *Monoclonal and Polyclonal Hypergammaglobulinemia – Clinical and Biological Significance*. Cambridge University Press.

6

Hypersensitivity

Since immunity was first recognized as a resistant state that followed infection, immunology developed primarily as an aspect of medical bacteriology with emphasis on acquired specific resistance to invasion by microorganisms as a means of protection against infection. Much of the present terminology originates from this early period in the development of immunology. The term immunity, meaning safe or exempt, has now been extended far beyond its early meaning and includes reactions to foreign material such as grafted tissues, blood products and various bland chemical substances none of which bears any relation to infectious agents. Some forms of immune reaction rather than providing exemption or safety to the affected individual can produce severe and occasionally fatal results. These are known as '**hypersensitivity reactions**' and in the main are due to tissue damage caused by effects of pharmacologically active agents such as histamine which are formed under certain conditions of antigen-antibody combination.

The term **allergy** was originally coined by von Pirquet early this century to describe the altered reactivity of an animal following exposure to a foreign antigen, and included both immunity and hypersensitivity. The term, however, has over the years become restricted to refer only to the hypersensitivity which may be associated with the development of the immune response to a foreign substance.

Immediate and delayed hypersensitivity
There are two main forms of hypersensitivity reaction: **immediate** and **delayed** (Fig. 6.1). The immediate or **antibody-mediated** form appears rapidly and depends on the production of pharmacologically active mediator substances activated by antigen-antibody interaction. The delayed or **cell-mediated** form appears more slowly (usually after 24 hours) and depends on immunologically activated lymphoid cells which, on reaction with antigen, appear to release substances known as lymphokines having

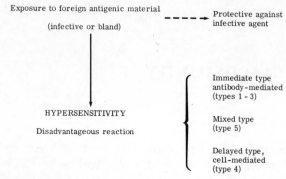

Fig. 6.1 Hypersensitivity reactions

a variety of effects on other cells and effects on blood vessel permeability (p. 74).

Various classifications of hypersensitivity reactions have been proposed and probably the most widely accepted is that of Coombs and Gell. This recognizes four types or categories of hypersensitivity reactions, three of which come under the heading of immediate antibody-mediated reactions: type 1, anaphylactic reactions; type 2, cytolytic or cytotoxic reactions; and type 3, toxic-complex syndrome. The fourth type is the cell-mediated delayed hypersensitivity form of reaction. An additional category is now recognized that is both antibody and cell-mediated and can be regarded as a **mixed** form of hypersensitivity. This is sometimes referred to as a type 5 reaction.

Anaphylactic reactions of type 1

If a guinea-pig is injected with a small dose of an antigen such as egg albumen no adverse effects are noted. If however, a second injection of the egg albumen antigen is given intravenously after an interval of about 10 days a condition known as 'anaphylactic shock' is likely to develop. The animal becomes restless, starts chewing and rubbing its nose with its front paws, respiration becomes laboured, the animal becomes cyanosed and may develop convulsions and die. The initial injection of antigen is termed the **sensitizing dose** and the second injection the **shocking dose**. During the interval between the two injections the animal has formed antibody and anaphylaxis is the result of interaction of the shocking dose of antigen with antibody which triggers the release of pharmacologically active substances causing increase in capillary permeability and contraction of smooth muscle in many parts of the body. In the guinea-pig this particularly affects the smooth muscles of the bronchioles causing respiratory embarrassment.

Pharmacological mediators. Four pharmacologically active substances have been implicated to varying degrees in anaphylactic reactions: (1) histamine, (2) 5-hydroxy-tryptamine, (3) slow-reacting substance, (4) the bradykinins. Predominant amongst these and responsible for many of the symptoms of anaphylactic shock is **histamine** which can be shown to be liberated *in vitro* when antibody-sensitized pieces of various tissues including uterine muscle, lung and intestine are exposed to contact with antigen. Sensitization may be produced by prior injection of antigen into the animal supplying the tissue which makes antibody as described above or the tissue may be sensitized passively by the addition of antibody produced in another animal. The typical contractions induced in this way in the uterus and intestine are called Schultze-Dale reactions after the originators. The histamine is derived from the granules of mast cells where it exists as its precursor histidine, in combination with heparin; these substances are released by the interaction of antigen with antibody via another pharmacologically active substance anaphylatoxin acting together with serum complement components (p. 19). The role of antibody in this reaction is considered on p. 96.

The eosinophil is thought to play an important part in anaphylactic reactions, many of these marrow-derived cells being found in the blood and tissues during an anaphylactic reaction. Eosinophils are attracted to the site of the reaction by an **eosinophil chemotactic factor** that is released following the interaction of antibody and antigen on the surface of a mast cell. The precise role of the eosinophil in anaphylactic reactions is not yet clear. Its suggested activities include the release of an inhibitor of histamine after having phagocytosed complexes of antibody and antigen and the repair of the tissue damage brought about in the hypersensitivity reaction. Eosinophil granules contain arylsulphatase, an enzyme that splits SRS-A into two inactive fragments and thus can control the smooth muscle spasm induced by SRS-A.

The other pharmacological mediators of immediate hypersensitivity reactions are: 5-hydroxy-tryptamine or serotonin which causes contraction of plain muscle and increased capillary permeability. It is of uncertain role in anaphylaxis, although it is probably involved in local intestinal food allergies; slow-reacting substance (or SRS-A) has a plain muscle contracting effect acting, unlike histamine, on the larger rather than smaller blood vessels.

SRS-A has a particularly marked bronchial constricting effect in man and is probably the predominant pharmacological agent in human asthma. Bradykinins are simple peptides formed from a plasma α globulin (kininogen) by plasma kinin-forming enzymes. They have histamine-like effects on smooth muscle and capillaries, and studies have shown that it is present in the blood stream in many species in the early stages of an anaphylactic reaction.

Systemic and local forms. In man there are two types of anaphylactic reaction – **systemic** and **local** – and which one of these develops depends on how the shocking dose of antigen enters the body. The systemic form of anaphylaxis is likely to develop if antigen is injected parenterally, as in the case of foreign serum (e.g. horse anti-tetanus serum), or a drug such as penicillin, or perhaps by the bite of an insect. The symptoms include dyspnoea with bronchospasm and laryngeal oedema, sometimes skin rashes, a fall in blood pressure and occasionally death. If, on the other hand, the antigen comes in contact with respiratory mucous membranes, then in a sensitized individual the local forms of anaphylaxis will develop – i.e. hay fever or asthma. If the intestinal mucous membrane of a susceptible individual comes in contact with the appropriate antigen (e.g. nuts, fish or strawberries), then a mixed form of reaction can develop with intestinal symptoms, skin rashes (urticaria) and sometimes the symptoms of asthma.

The antibodies involved in anaphylactic reactions
The role of IgE. In the human the antibodies which sensitize the tissues for anaphylactic reactions have been known for many years as **reaginic** antibodies. These antibodies have a strong affinity for tissues (cytotrophic) and can readily be detected in the serum of a sensitized individual by injecting a small quantity of the serum into the skin of a normal recipient, and 24 to 48 hours later, introducing the appropriate antigen into the injection site. Within about 20 minutes a weal and flare erythematous reaction develops at the injection site, just like the response to an injection of histamine. This reaction is called the P.K. test after its originators Prausnitz and Küstner.

The nature of reaginic antibody was not finally elucidated until late in 1967 when a hitherto undescribed form of myeloma protein was discovered in Sweden although work in America suggested the existence of an immunoglobulin distinct from IgG, IgM or IgA. This made it possible (using an antiserum prepared in a sheep to the myeloma globulin) to show in normal human serum a new class of immunoglobulin present in very low concentration (10–130 μg/100 ml of serum cf. 900–1800 mg of IgG/100 ml serum). The skin sensitizing activity of reaginic antibody could readily be neutralized by means of the antiserum to this new immunoglobulin which has been named IgE (p. 48). The concentration of IgE in patients with allergic asthma has been found to be much higher than in normal individuals although the level of IgE in the circulation does not correlate with the severity of the allergic symptoms. The comparatively low levels of IgE found in serum presumably reflect the affinity of this immunoglobulin for tissues so that freshly made IgE is very soon removed from serum when it comes in contact with the appropriate cell receptors on mast cells and possibly elsewhere.

IgE appears to have four main activities: (1) the capacity to bind via its Fc fragment to mast cells in basophils; (2) subsequent interaction with antigen that takes place on the cell membrane of the mast cell; (3) resultant triggering of the release of pharmacological mediators; (4) attraction of other cell types–eosinophils. The third of these activities, namely the triggering of the release of pharmacological mediators from mast cells, has been the subject of much recent study and it appears that two adjacent molecules of IgE (attached to Fc receptors on mast cells) must be **bridged** by antigen before degranulation takes place. Monovalent antigens (i.e., with a single antigenic determinant) will block the IgE antibody from further interaction with antigen but will **not** trigger degranulation. The triggering appears to follow the entry of calcium ions into the mast cell, presumably as part of the membrane changes that finally lead to the degranulation or exocytosis process.

Immunological approaches to the prevention of anaphylaxis
Blocking antibody. On consideration of the mechanism of systemic anaphylaxis it would seem likely that if the parenterally injected antigen could be prevented from reaching the tissue-fixed IgE then anaphylaxis would not develop. This desirable state of affairs can be achieved by the simple expedient of injecting frequent small doses of the antigen to which the patient is sensitized. This induces the formation of increasing levels of IgG antibody which, circulating in the blood and tissue fluids, mops up the injected antigen so that it does not reach the tissue-fixed IgE (Fig. 6.2). This IgG antibody has been termed **blocking antibody** and its induction is the basis of desensitization treatment in allergic individuals. As might be expected this method is much more effective in preventing systemic anaphylactic reactions than the local forms where the antigen does

ANAPHYLAXIS (Type 1)

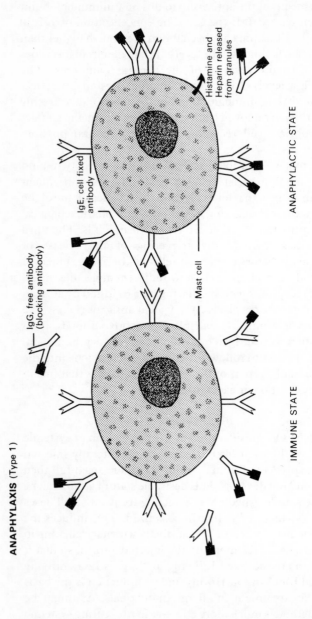

IgG, free antibody (blocking antibody)

IgE, cell fixed antibody

Histamine and Heparin released from granules

Mast cell

IMMUNE STATE

ANAPHYLACTIC STATE

Antigen molecule   Immunoglobulin molecule

Fig. 6.2 Diagrammatic view of the possible difference between an 'immune state' (i.e. when immunized animal will not develop anaphylaxis on challenge with antigen) and an 'anaphylactic state'. Here there is insufficient antibody free in the tissue fluids to mop up the antigen thus allowing it to combine with reaginic antibody (IgE) attached to cell. The interaction triggers the release of histamine and heparin from mast cell granules.

not enter the blood stream. To prevent local anaphylaxis the blocking antibody would need to be present in the mucous secretions and parenteral injection of antigen is hardly the best way to achieve this (see p. 125 for discussion of immunization against influenza virus).

In theory it should be possible by raising the level of IgE to antigens other than those responsible for the allergic sensitization to occupy the tissue receptors by non-specific IgE antibodies rather than those formed to the sensitizing antigen. Whether such a procedure is feasible remains to be established. Recent work using rats sensitized to benzylpenicilloyl (a penicillin derivative) raises the possibility that B cell tolerance can be induced to the antigen by repeated injections (subcutaneously or intraperitoneally) of the benzylpenicilloyl linked to a carrier, a random polymer of glutamic acid and lysine (D–GL). Levels of IgE and IgG to the penicillin derivative are markedly reduced for at least six months.

For pollen or seasonal allergies desensitizing injections are given before the onset of the pollen season and about 70 per cent of cases obtain clinical benefit from the treatment, and with ragweed antigen marked increases in the ratio of blocking IgG to IgE levels have recently been found.

Symptomatic treatment of allergies commonly involves the use of anti-histamines and more recently disodium cromoglycate has come into use which is effective in blocking histamine release if the drug is present before challenge with antigen. Isoprenaline and theophylline, which increase the level of intracellular cyclic-AMP, in turn reduces histamine release from mast cells. Cortico steroids also have a beneficial effect in type 1 allergic disorders, although their mode of action is unclear.

Cytolytic or cytotoxic (type 2) reactions

Cell-associated antigens. Reactions of this type are initiated by an antigenic component either part of a tissue cell or closely associated with it (e.g. a drug attached to the cell wall (Fig. 6.3). The antibodies directed against such a cell-associated antigen bring about a cytotoxic or cytolytic effect usually involving complement. Reactions of this type include the cytolytic effect of anti-red cell antibodies, induced by incompatible blood transfusion, on the foreign erythrocytes. Haemolytic disease of the newborn has a similar mechanism as do certain forms of auto-immune haemolytic anaemia in which the patient forms antibodies against autologous red cells. There are many examples of these cytotoxic or cytolytic reactions which are brought about by an immune reaction to a

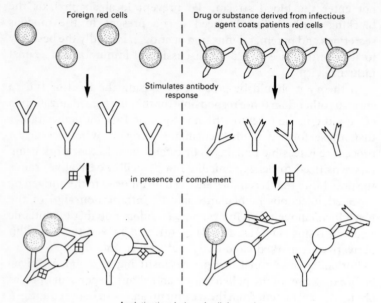

Fig. 6.3 Cytolytic and cytotoxic (type 2) reactions.

foreign substance which becomes attached to the cell membranes of erythrocytes, leucocytes or platelets. One of the best known examples of this phenomenon is Sedormid (apronal) purpura. The complexing of the drug Sedormid with platelets results in an antibody response directed against the platelet-adsorbed drug which brings about destruction of the platelets and purpura. As a result of the elucidation of the mechanism of this disease by Ackroyd in London, Sedormid has been withdrawn from use. This type of reaction may be more widespread than is generally suspected. A variety of infectious diseases due to salmonella organisms and mycobacteria are associated with haemolytic anaemia, and there is evidence, particularly in studies in salmonella infections, that the haemolysis is due to an immune reaction against a lipopolysaccharide bacterial endotoxin which becomes coated on to the patient's erythrocytes. A detailed study of *Salmonella gallinarum* infection in chickens has shown conclusively that the red cells are coated, have a shorter life in the circulation due to haemolysis and that the development of haemolysis directly parallels the level of the anti-lipopolysaccharide antibody.

Toxic-complex syndrome (type 3) reactions
Serum sickness and Arthus reactions. These reactions are due to the

combination of antigen with circulating antibody with the formation of microprecipitates in and around small blood vessels causing inflammation and sometimes mechanical blocking of these vessels which results in interference with the blood supply to surrounding tissues. There are two types of reaction which fall into this category: **serum sickness** which is a systemic form and the **Arthus reaction** which is a local form.

Serum sickness develops, as the name suggests, in individuals injected with foreign serum and was described soon after the introduction of parenteral administration, for therapeutic purposes, of diphtheria antitoxin prepared in the horse. Foreign serum protein is eliminated from the circulation over a period of a few weeks and after the injection of 10 to 20 ml there will still be a large amount present by the time an immune response to the foreign serum protein develops. This results in the formation of antibody-antigen complexes that can cause a wide variety of symptoms ranging from anaphylactic reactions such as asthma or laryngeal oedema when IgE antibody attached to mast cells is involved, to symptoms dependent on the deposition of immune complexes (antigen + IgG antibody) in blood vessels where they activate complement and cause inflammatory changes. Fixation of the first component of complement C (p. 16) leads to the formation of anaphylatoxin involved in histamine release. The inflammatory cells are mainly polymorphs attracted by the trimolar C567 complex that has chemotactic activity. Proteolytic enzymes released by polymorphs damage adjacent tissues and plasma kinins are also activated. The intensity of the reaction depends upon the concentration of complexes and on the ability of the antibody to activate complement. IgM, IgG1, IgG2 and IgG3 antibodies have this ability (p. 55) whereas IgG4, IgA and IgE do not. The clinical manifestations depend upon where the immune complexes form or lodge.

On the basis of experimental work in rabbits two forms of reaction have been recognized: (1) following a single large dose of antigen which results in arthritis, glomerulonephritis and coronary artery vasculitis; (2) following daily doses of antigen which results after a few weeks in glomerulonephritis. The first form is complement dependent whereas the second occurs even in complement depleted animals. The first form of reaction in humans manifests itself by affecting the kidneys with the development of glomerulonephritis and in severe cases renal failure, the heart, with myocarditis and valvulitis, and the joints which become swollen and painful. Urticaria sometimes develops and the patient becomes pyrexial. The symptoms disappear whenever all the foreign serum protein is eliminated.

Antigens other than serum proteins can cause serum sickness. Nowadays the most likely causes are drugs such as penicillin and sulphonamides. The susceptible patient will develop rashes (urticarial, morbilliform or scarlatinoform), pyrexia, arthralgia, lymphadenopathy and perhaps nephritis some 8 to 12 days after giving the drug. It seems likely that many bacterial infections and some virus ones, include development of hypersensitivity of this type, as rashes, joint pains and sometimes mild haematuria are not uncommon. In poststreptococcal glomerulonephritis streptococcal antigens have been detected in the glomeruli (see also p. 145). In virus hepatitis circulating immune complexes have been found associated with periarteritis nodosa. Many of the clinical features of the autoimmune disease systemic lupus erythematosus (discussed on p. 147) appear to result from arteritis, and deposits of immunoglobulin and complement (probably complexed with DNA) have been found in the skin lesions and glomeruli of patients with the disease.

The Arthus reaction like serum sickness is brought about by the formation of antibody-antigen complexes but in this case the phenomenon is a local one at the site of injection of antigen. The Arthus reaction occurs in walls of small blood vessels in the presence of large quantities of IgG antibody forming microprecipitates with antigen. The resulting vasculitis develops a few hours after injection of antigen and persists for 12 to 24 hours. Immune complexes can be shown microscopically in the vessel wall using the fluorescent antibody technique (p. 185) and there is a massive infiltration of granulocytes brought about by a chemotactic effect generated by the antigen-antibody complex. There is activation of the vasoactive amines such as histamine, with resulting increase in vascular permeability and consequent oedema. These reactions may occur in diabetics who have received many injections of insulin and have developed high levels of IgG antibody to antigenic constituents in the insulin preparation.

Arthus reactions in the bronchial or alveolar wall may explain the late asthmatic reactions that occur 7 to 8 hours after inhalation of antigen. These may be of particular importance in the 'allergic alveolitis' seen in farmers sensitive to mouldy hay antigen (see page 134) and maltworkers sensitive to *Aspergillus clavatus* of contaminated barley. In some cases of tuberculosis, sarcoidosis, leprosy and streptococcal infections, vascular inflammatory lesions are seen mainly in the legs. These are variously referred to as erythema nodosum, nodular vasculitis and erythema induratum and may be due to the deposition of immune complexes and the development of an Arthus reaction.

Delayed hypersensitivity (type 4) cell-mediated hypersensitivity

Lymphocyte-mediated reactions and 'lymphokines'. These can be defined as specifically provoked, slowly evolving (24 to 48 hours) mixed cellular reactions involving particularly lymphocytes and macrophages. The reaction is not brought about by circulating antibody but by sensitized lymphoid cells and can be transferred in experimental animals by means of such cells but not serum. The classical example of this type of reaction is the tuberculin response which has over the years received detailed study. To induce this response a tuberculin-sensitized individual is given an intradermal injection of 0.1 ml of a 1 in 1000 dilution of a protein extract of tubercle bacilli (purified protein derivative PPD). An indurated inflammatory reaction in the skin, measuring a few millimetres in diameter, appears about 24 hours later and persists for a few weeks. In the human the injection site is infiltrated with large numbers of mononuclear cells, mainly lymphocytes, with about 10–20 per cent macrophages. Most of these cells are in and around small blood vessels. Despite intensive investigation of the delayed hypersensitivity reaction immunologists are far from understanding the mechanisms underlying this phenomenon. A possible explanation is that amongst the continuous traffic of lymphocytes passing through the tissues (p. 82) there are some sensitized cells possibly with 'antibody-like receptors' on their surface. These cells interact with antigen they meet and in some unknown way influence other lymphocytes and phagocytes to migrate to the area.

In the last few years a group of as yet ill-defined substances have been shown to be released by lymphocytes coming in contact with the antigen to which they have been sensitized. The name **lymphokines** has been proposed to describe this group of non-antibody lymphocyte factors. They are discussed on page 74 and Table 4.6 shows the range of factors produced. Their main role appears to be to **recruit** non-sensitized (uncommitted) lymphoid cells to the site of inflammation and to **retain** them at the site where they become activated, thus **amplifying** the immune response. An important factor appears to be responsible for inducing proliferation of lymphocytes at the site of localization and has been termed mitogenic factor. A cytotoxic effect has been demonstrated in tissue culture experiments affecting lymphocytes and other cells (lymphotoxin). The best known of the lymphokines is the macrophage migration inhibition factor. This effect is readily demonstrated *in vitro* using peritoneal exudate cells from an animal sensitized to an antigen such as tuberculin. The peritoneal exudate cells which are mainly macrophages are collected in a capillary tube that is placed on a glass coverslip in a small tissue culture chamber (Fig. 4.17). After 24 hours macrophages show a fan-shaped area of migration around the end of the capillary tube. If however, the tuberculin antigen is placed in the tissue culture medium no migration occurs. The effect appears to be due to the release, from the small number of lymphocytes in peritoneal exudate, of a lymphokine known as macrophage migration inhibition factor or MIF. The specificity of the reaction has been shown with several other antigens including bovine gamma globulin, histoplasmin and dinitrophenol. The MIF appears to be released from cells concerned with the cell-mediated immune state rather than cells concerned with making humoral antibody. The chemical nature of MIF has not yet been established although it appears in guinea pigs to have an MW of 35–50,000 (like some of the other lymphokines) and is likely to be glycoprotein. *In vivo* the factor may be responsible for the formation of large aggregates of macrophages in the lymphoid tissues (and perhaps elsewhere), although like the other lymphokines the precise role of MIF in delayed hypersensitivity reaction is not yet clear and much further work is required to separate and identify the nature and functional activities of the various substances involved. Whether or not macrophages in delayed hypersensitivity reaction sites contribute lysosomal enzymes from their intracellular granules thus bringing about further inflammatory changes has yet to be determined.

Inducing agents. Delayed hypersensitivity reactions are characteristically induced by intracellular infectious agents including salmonellae, brucellae, streptococci and a wide range of viruses including measles and mumps viruses, vaccinia and herpes simplex (see also p. 127). Those with most clinical relevance are reactions due to vaccinia – the so-called 'reaction of immunity' occurring 24 to 72 hours after vaccination. This reaction does not proceed like a primary vaccination through the pustular stage and leaves no scar but instead has all the features of a delayed hypersensitivity reaction. The other important reaction is the 'pseudo-Schick' response occurring within 24 hours after the intradermal injection of diphtheria toxoid. This delayed response disappears within six days and also affects the control injected site (heat-treated toxoid). Delayed hypersensitivity reactions sometimes develop following sensitization to a variety of metals such as nickel and chromium, to simple chemical substances such as dyestuffs, potassium dichromate (affecting cement workers), primulin from primula plants, poison ivy and chemicals such as picryl chloride, dinitrochlorobenzene, and paraphenylene diamine (from hair dyes). Penicillin sensitization is a common clinical complication following the topical application of the antibiotic in ointments or creams. These substances are not themselves antigenic and only become so on combination by covalent bonds with proteins in the skin. The clinical symptoms induced in these 'contact hypersensitivity' reactions (contact dermatitis) include redness, swelling, vesicles, scaling and exudation of fluid.

It is conceivable that, in future, use may be made of the delayed hypersensitivity response in the treatment of tumours. Some recent experiments in man show that certain skin tumours, if painted with a simple chemical antigen as described above, underwent a marked hypersensitivity reaction and then healed with the disappearance of the tumour. One explanation of the effect is that the lymphokine – lymphotoxin – is released during the hypersensitivity reaction and destroys the tumour cells. Much more work is clearly required before this can be regarded as a useful clinical procedure (see also p. 169).

Antibody-dependent cell-mediated cytotoxicity

This mixed form of hypersensitivity sometimes called type 5 reactions is mediated by at least two distinct types of non-immune cells acting in conjunction with antibody directed at a target cell.

The non-immune 'killer' cells (or K cells) take two forms:

1. Cells morphologically similar to small or medium-sized lymphocytes without easily demonstrable immunoglobulin on their surface that are not glass adherent (in contrast to macrophages) or phagocytic. They are prominent in human peripheral blood and have receptors for the Fc portion of IgG and sometimes for products of C3. It is believed that these cells are cytotoxic for antibody coated tumour cells (e.g. melanoma cells) and for virus infected cells (e.g. herpes simplex infected cells).

2. A glass adherent cell (possibly a monocyte) that lyses antibody coated red blood cells. This form of lysis takes place without involving the complement system.

These mixed forms of hypersensitivity reaction can readily be demonstrated *in vitro* and there a a number of reports showing cytotoxic effects against various antibody-coated target cells including human tissue cells in certain 'auto-immune' disease states (see chap. 9). Whether or not this mixed form of hypersensitivity has its *in vivo* counterpart remains to be established.

FURTHER READING

Austen, F. J. & Block, K. J. (1972) *Biochemistry of Acute Allergic Reactions*. Oxford: Blackwell.

Brostoff, J. (1973) Atopic allergy. *Brit. J. hosp. Med.*, **9,** 29.

Cream, J. J. (1973) Immune complex diseases. *Brit. J. hosp. Med.*, **9,** 8.

Cochrane, C. G., Koffler, D. (1973) Immune complex disease in experimental animals and man. *Adv. Immunol.*, **18,** 185.

Gell, P. G. H., Coombs, R. R. A. & Lachmann, P. J. (1975) *Clinical Aspects of Immunology*. 3rd edition. Oxford: Blackwell.

Turk, J. L. (1967) Delayed hypersensitivity. In *Frontiers in Biology*, Vol. 4, ed. Neuberger, A. & Tatum, E. L. Amsterdam: North Holland.

Turk, J. L. (1967) Delayed hypersensitivity – specific cell-mediated immunity. *Br. med. Bull.*, **23,** No. 1.

Turk, J. L. (1969) *Immunology in Clinical Medicine*. London: Heinemann.

Uhr, J. W. (1966) Delayed hypersensitivity. *Physiol. Rev.*, **46,** 359.

7

The immunology of tissue transplantation

The tissue cells of animals contain antigens that are specific for the species of origin of the cell, and which if implanted into an animal of another species will induce an immune response. This response rapidly destroys the implanted cells and has the characteristics of the primary and secondary immune response as already described for antigens in general. In addition to species specific antigens, differences also exist between individual members of the same species so that transfer of tissue cells between members induces a similar immune reaction. The closer the relationship between two individuals of the same species the more likely are implanted cells to survive and in the case of identical twins survival is assured. Inbred strains of animals, particularly mice, have been developed which are genetically identical and these are widely used in experimental work on tissue transplantation immunology.

In man surgical techniques are available to enable transplantation of many organs and tissues but unfortunately a high proportion of organ transplants fail because of rejection by the immune response or because of the side effects of attempts to suppress the immune response, due to toxicity of the drugs or their depressive effect on resistance to infection.

Table 7.1 Transplantation terminology (older terminology in brackets)

Relationship between donor and recipient	Term applied to relationship	Prefix applied to graft, antigen or antibody
Of different species	Xenogeneic (heterogeneic)	Xeno- (hetero-)
Of same species but different genetic constitution	Allogeneic (homologous)	Allo- (homo-)
Of same inbred strain	Syngeneic (isogeneic) (isologous)	—
Same individual	Autologous	Auto-

Transplantation antigen systems

The first systematic studies on the antigens carried by cells which determine whether a graft will be rejected or not were carried out in inbred strains of mice of known genetic make up.

It was found that there were very many antigenic differences between tissues of different strains of mice, the number of separate antigens involved being estimated at between 15 and 500 in different experiments. However, it was found that, just as in the red cell antigenic system, some antigens were very 'strong' and others very weak. The strong transplantation or 'histocompatibility' antigens of the mouse are controlled by the H-2 genetic locus and in man by the HLA locus.

The mouse H-2 system appears to consist of a system of closely linked genes and there are hundreds of possible combinations resulting in different H-2 antigens. H-2 antigens are found in large amounts in epithelium and lymphoid tissues, in very small amounts in kidney or muscle and are virtually absent from brain and testis.

In man, two strong and several weak histocompatibility systems have been found. As mentioned already the HLA is the strong system with the ABH blood group system next in importance. The major loci are very complex, the antigens being determined by a chromosomal region rather than by a single gentic locus.

Chemical studies on soluble H-2 antigens have shown them to be glycoproteins. Analysis of the amino acid constitution of extracted transplantation antigen of two different inbred strains of guinea-pig indicates that they are distinct.

Leucocyte grouping. The strong antigens of the HLA system are widely distributed in the tissues but absent from the red blood cells which contain only the ABH antigens.

Fortunately blood leucocytes carry all the known HLA antigens and it is therefore possible to test for the presence or absence of antigens of the system using leucocyte agglutination and cytotoxicity tests (p. 187). In principle the leuco-agglutination test is performed with leucocytes separated from the erythrocytes of anticoagulant-treated blood. Specific antisera for HLA antigens are then used to agglutinate the leucocytes and the tests are read under the microscope. The cytotoxic test is carried out with a purified suspension of blood lymphocytes which are mixed with antisera to HLA antigens in the presence of complement (p. 187). If the lymphocytes carry the appropriate antigens the antiserum will combine and in the presence of complement will damage the cell membrane. The resulting increased cell membrane permeability is usually detected by dye uptake into the cell.

Despite the very great diversity among HLA alleles of unrelated subjects it is encouraging to find that about a third of kidneys from unrelated donors survive for a year or longer although only a third of them show normal kidney function. Although this partial success must be dependent to an extent on the use of immunosuppressive agents, differences in the 'strength' of individual HLA antigens is probably partly responsible.

Mechanisms of graft rejection

There are two main types of graft rejection process: (a) the so-called 'first set' response which occurs about 10 days after a first graft from

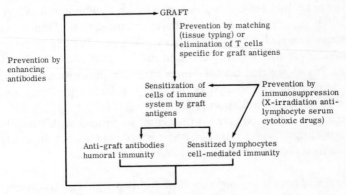

Fig. 7.1 Schematic view of rejection mechanisms and their prevention.

an unrelated donor, (b) the 'second set' response occurring in about 7 days in an animal which had previously received a graft from the same unrelated donor. This phenomenon of first and second set rejection can be compared to primary and secondary immunization – the accelerated secondary response being brought about by stimulation of an already sensitized or 'primed' immune system.

The role of lymphoid cells. It can be shown histologically that grafts undergoing rejection are heavily infiltrated with lymphocytes and that there is extensive vascular damage. Other types of cell of the immune system, such as plasma cells and macrophages, are also frequently found in association with graft rejection. The ability to reject grafts can readily be transferred from one animal to another by a process known as **adoptive transfer** of lymphoid cells from an immune animal (i.e. one capable of a second set graft rejection) to a non-immune recipient of the same strain. Lymphoid cells appear to be able to transfer this ability most effectively when taken before the circulating antibody level reaches its peak. Contrary to expectation, it is possible to show, using isotope-labelled cells, that it is not the transferred cells which migrate to the graft but those of the recipient, the donated cells in the main homing to the lymphoid organs, as no more are found in the graft than at control sites. It is, however, possible that those few donated cells which settle in the graft area are cells specifically sensitized to the graft antigens whilst those settling out elsewhere are the unsensitized cells. From what is known about the recirculating lymphocyte pool (p. 82) it seems likely that there is a good chance of cells with a specific ability to react to an antigen, coming in contact with such material in a graft during the process of lymphocyte recirculation. Donor lymphocytes carried over as 'passengers' in the vascular bed of the graft could be a source of transplantation antigens that could sensitize the host. In rats pretreatment of donors with immunosuppressive agents to deplete the lymphocyte population resulted in prolongation of graft survival. Stimulation of the host cells residing in the lymphoid organs would be expected if they came in contact with transplantation antigens carried by passenger lymphocytes from the graft, as described above, which themselves reach the spleen.

The role of circulating antibody. The ability to reject grafts cannot be transferred from one animal to another by means of passively injected antibody. This does not rule out the possibility that antibody can play a part in graft rejection, because when the serum, containing at best about 1 per cent specific antibody, is injected into a recipient the diluting effect of the blood and tissue fluids considerably reduces the possibility of the antibody reaching the graft site in an adequate concentration to influence the viability of the graft. The same antibody-containing serum can readily be shown *in vitro* to be cytotoxic, in the presence of complement, for cells containing antigens to which the antibody was produced. However, this is an artificial situation and does not take into account the dilution effects discussed above. Kidney grafts which have survived for some time, perhaps months or years, can, it seems, be rejected by serum antibody alone without any evidence of invasion of the graft by lymphoid cells. Deposits of immunoglobulin and complement can be detected particularly in the walls of blood vessels. Although at this stage no antibodies may be detected in the serum, if the rejected kidney is removed they soon appear, suggesting that the antibodies were rapidly removed by combination with kidney antigens. The kidney is rejected by the development of a progressive vasculitis affecting glomerular and other vessels. Attempts have been made to recover antibody by elution from rejected kidneys removed from 27 patients. Seven of the kidneys contained recoverable antibody and this often differed from that found in the patients serum supporting the view that grafted incompatible kidneys filter out antibody from the circulation.

Locally produced antibody and non-antibody lymphocyte factors. The possibility is quite strong that antibody made locally in a graft by the infiltrating lymphoid cells is present in a sufficiently high concentration in the area immediately surrounding the antibody-producing cell to damage incompatible cells of the graft. This situation can be compared to the observation made *in vitro* with the Jerne plaque technique (p. 41) in which lymphocytes can be shown to be producing antibody to sheep red blood cells which produces a surrounding halo of lysis of the red cells in the presence of complement. Indeed, lymphocytes and plasma cells invading grafts can be shown to contain immunoglobulin. Evidence that immunoglobulin is combining with antigen during graft rejection is provided by a detectable fall in the serum complement level. There are a number of other possible direct ways in which the infiltrating lymphocytes can influence survival of the graft: (a) the antibody which they produce may activate the various pharmacological mediators of immediate hypersensitivity reactions such as histamine (p. 95) and these will bring about changes in the vessels of the graft; (b) the lymphocytes on contact with antigen may release macrophage migration inhibition factor (MIF) (p. 74) which will cause accumulation of macrophages in the graft; (c) it is known that sensitized lymphocytes can influence non-immune lymphocytes to behave aggressively towards cells in their vicinity and induce cytotoxic effects. How this is brought about is not clear but may conceivably depend upon the release of one of the factors mentioned above.

It can thus be seen that the reaction against a graft depends upon a complex series of interrelated phenomena some of which are specifically induced by the foreign nature of graft antigens. Other phenomena are non-specific in the immunological sense and occur as part of an inflammatory process.

Immunosuppression

Graft rejection, as has been noted, involves a sequence of separate phenomena developing from initial contact of the foreign antigens with the host immunological system through to rejection itself. The steps include establishment of lymphatic drainage, antigen release, its contact with cells of the immune system, proliferation of antibody-forming cells of the lymphoid tissues, the inflammatory response and release of pharmacological mediators and cytotoxic effects of lymphoid cells and/or antibody on the graft tissues.

Prevention of sensitization; tolerance to graft antigens. Interference with any of these stages would be likely to interfere with the rejection process. One of the most interesting approaches, which is as yet unfortunately only at the experimental stage, is interference with what might be termed the afferent arc of the process of rejection, namely the initial sensitization of the lymphoid cells. If it were possible to induce immune tolerance (p. 64) to the strong histocompatibility antigens of tissue grafts, then clearly immunological rejection would not take place. The tolerant animal although unable to react against the antigen to which it is tolerant can still respond to other antigens such as potentially infective agents like bacteria, fungi or viruses; this obviates one of the greatest difficulties associated with immunosuppressive procedures.

As has been noted earlier, Mitchison (using serum protein antigens) has shown that there are two types of tolerance, so-called 'high dose' tolerance where the immune system is overloaded with excess antigen, and 'low dose' tolerance where only minute quantities of antigen are administered. Although the molecular processes underlying these phenomena are not as yet understood, clearly the 'low dose' tolerance phenomenon has great potential application to transplantation problems. When it becomes possible to extract purified transplantation antigens from tissue, it should then be possible to prepare an individual for graft acceptance by inducing low dose tolerance to the appropriate antigens.

Some progress has been made recently in the induction of specific tolerance against transplantation antigens in rats by eliminating the T lymphocytes which normally respond to graft antigens. It has been done by preparing antibodies against the T cell receptors for the major histocompatibility antigen. This is achieved by mating two inbred strains of rat: the hybrids would express the histocompatibility antigens of each parent and thus be tolerant to them. The implication is that the T cells would not express receptors for the antigens whilst each of the parents would express receptors for the histocompatibility antigens of the other strain. Thus by injecting the hybrid rats with lymphocytes from a parent the hybrids would not react to the histocompatibility antigen but would react to the receptors for the antigen on the parental cells.

T lymphocytes shed their receptors and it is therefore possible to extract these for the major histocompatibility antigen by binding them to the antibody (attached to an inert particle). The purified T cell receptors are then chemically modified by cross linking with gluteraldehyde (to make them immunogenic) and when injected into an inbred strain of rats (Lewis) with adjuvant, are able to slow down the rejection of grafts from another inbred strain (DA). The eventual rejection of the graft in 24 days (compared to 11 days in untreated rats) is probably due to minor histocompatibility differences. The prolongation of graft survival is likely to be due to suppression or elimination of lymphocytes bearing the receptor for the major histocompatibility antigen by the antibodies induced by the chemically modified purified receptor.

Another approach at inducing transplantation tolerance is the repeated injection of massive doses of serum into neonatal rats. The serum contains small amounts of histocompatibility antigen and this is sufficient in neonatal rats to induce a lasting tolerance to certain skin grafts showing strong histocompatibility differences between donor and recipient. The practical value of this approach is clearly limited by the requirement that tolerance be induced in neonatal animals.

Immunological enhancement. Another phenomenon relevant to the maintenance of incompatible grafts is 'immunological enhancement'. This is brought about by antibody produced against graft antigens that can under certain circumstances protect the graft from attack by cells of the immune system. This system has been used successfully in rats with incompatible kidney grafts, the animals being previously immunized with tissue from the prospective donor. The grafts exhibit normal renal function for a year or more afterwards. The method has been applied in a few instances to human kidney grafts and the results suggest that the method may be of considerable future value. The mechanism may involve coating of the cells of the graft by non-complement-fixing antibody and/or direct inhibition of antibody production against the graft brought about by the antibody. The danger of the antibody damaging the graft will require the use of antisera (directed against the histocompatibility antigen) that has been treated so as to eliminate any cytotoxic effects. This could be achieved by making use of antibody fragments (Fab) that do not bind complement (p. 49).

Practical approaches. In practice there are at the moment three main approaches to the problem of immunosuppression: (1) X-irradiation to knock out the lymphoid tissues and abolish the immune response; (2) immuno-suppressive drugs – antimetabolites and anti-inflammatory agents to prevent proliferation of antibody-forming cells; (3) immunological methods – anti-lymphocyte serum (ALS) produced, for example, in the horse, to attack the lymphocytes directly and destroy them before they attack the graft.

Whole body X-irradiation used in the early days of organ transplantation has been replaced in the main by immunosuppressive drugs and ALS. Some attention has been given to reducing the lymphocyte count in the peripheral blood by passing it through an extracorporeal shunt and irradiating it outside the body. This method although tried so far only on a small scale and with a limited degree of success may perhaps, with development, become of value in the future. The drugs prednisone and Imuran (azathioprine) in combination are widely used and for immunosuppression are often given together with ALS. These substances in high dosage are toxic but haemodialysis before operation and during rejection crises reduces their toxicity in renal transplant cases.

Any of these regimes clearly carries with it the considerable risk of infection and the commonest cause of death after kidney grafting is not graft rejection but infection with fungi, viruses and bacteria. Another apparent complication noted in the last few years is the small but significant increase in reticulosarcomata following prolonged immunosuppressive therapy. This could conceivably be due to inhibition of the immunological surveillance mechanism (chap. 11).

Anti-lymphocyte serum has the advantage of primarily affecting the thymus-dependent lymphocytes of the spleen and lymph nodes, and lymphocytes circulating in the blood. This results in a suppression of the cell-mediated immune response with only a slight effect on the circulating antibody response. Thus, whilst suppressing the graft rejection mechanisms ALS leaves the animal able to produce circulating antibody against infecting microorganisms and their products. However, infections caused by intracellular agents such as virus in which protection depends on cell-mediated immunity (p. 127) still remain a possible complication in this form of immunosuppression and different preparations of ALS may vary in their effect on the antibody response. Furthermore, ALS can destroy platelets because of shared platelet and leucocyte antigen and may require prior absorption with platelet suspensions. Anaphylactic reactions may occur because of the foreign nature of the protein and severe pain frequently occurs at the injection site.

The possibility arises that in the future the immune response to histocompatibility antigens may conceivably be prevented by giving passive antibody against the transplantation antigens in the same way as can rhesus immunization (p. 158).

FURTHER READING

Bagshawe, K. D. (1972) Immunosuppression. Brit. J. hosp. Med., 8, 677.

Berenbaum, M. C. (1967) Transplantation and immunosuppression. In Modern Trends in Immunology, 2, p. 292, ed. Cruickshank, R. & Weir, D. M. London: Butterworth.

James, K. (1967) Anti-lymphocyte antibody: a review. Clin. exp. Immun., 2, 615.

Merrill, J. P. (1967) Human tissue transplantation. Adv. Immun., 2, 615.

Perkins, H. A. (1976) Transplantation immunology. In Basic and Clinical Immunology, eds. Fudenberg, H. H., Stites, D. P., Caldwell, J. L. & Wells, J. V. Los Altos: Lange.

Porter, K. A. (1967) Symposium on tissue and organ transplantation. J. clin. Path., Suppl. 20, 415.

Rapaport, F. T. & Dausset, J. (1968) Human Transplantation. New York: Grune & Stratton.

Roberts, C. J. (1972) Transplantation immunity. Brit. J. hosp. Med., 8, 695.

8

Infection, immunity and protection

Earlier chapters of this book deal with the mechanisms and characteristics of acquired immunity, both cell-mediated and humoral, and with the interactions between antibody and antigen resulting for example in the lysis by complement of microorganisms. It is necessary, however, to stress that neither the production of antibody to the antigens of an invading microorganism, nor even the combination of the antibody with such antigen, is in itself any guarantee that the infective agent will be inactivated or eliminated from the body.

Evasion
Microorganisms have numerous ways of protecting themselves from, and sidetracking, the immune reactions of the host. For example, the pneumococcus secretes large quantities of capsular polysaccharide that repels phagocytes and mops up antibody as it is produced, thus allowing the pneumococcus itself to proliferate unhindered. Trypanosomes appear to change their surface antigenic make-up from one generation to the next, so that the antibody made in response to the antigens of the original organism is inactive against the second generation of organisms. Many microorganisms, particularly tubercle bacilli, brucellae and many viruses, disappear inside tissue cells before sufficient antibody is produced to act against them. It has in the last few years been found that leprosy bacilli, which are similar in many ways to tubercle bacilli, have the ability to destroy the cells in the thymus-dependent areas of the lymphoid tissues. This prevents the mounting of a cell-mediated immune response (p. 71) against the invading organisms and allows its unhindered proliferation. The same appears to be true for cutaneous leishmaniasis where instances have been described of a loss of cell-mediated immunity. In short, a particular microorganism is pathogenic because in some way it is able to circumvent at least initially, the immune mechanisms of the host. In a situation where the host immune defence mechanisms are defective in some

way (often called the compromised host) then the distinction between pathogenic and non-pathogenic microorganisms becomes unimportant. All microorganisms that are human parasites have the capacity to produce infection in such a defective host. The breakdown of the normal host-parasite relationship then assumes central importance. Restoration of normal immune function is likely to be of more importance in the recovery of the patient than specific antimicrobial drug treatment.

The host immune mechanisms may be **compromised** in a large number of different ways, for example, in defects of humoral or cell-mediated immunity (congenital or acquired); depressed numbers or, functioning of polymorpho nuclear leucocytes; after splenectomy; after X-rays or immunosuppressive drugs; after implantation of foreign bodies (heart valves, catheters); after burn injury.

Epithelial attachment and infection

The attachment of a microorganism to an epithelial surface is a prerequisite for the development of an infectious process (excluding entry at sites of trauma). The mucosal surfaces of the respiratory, intestinal and genitourinary tracts are of primary

Table 8.1 Some examples of the ways in which microorganisms can sidetrack the immune mechanisms

Microorganism	Method of evasion
Pneumococcus	Capsular polysaccharide mops up antibody and prevents opsonization
Virulent strains of *Staph. aureus*	Anti-inflammatory factor limiting increased vascular permeability and access of antibody, complement and cells
Intracellular organisms (e.g. tubercle bacilli, brucellae viruses, leprosy bacilli,	Intracellular localization prevents access of protective antibody
Certain viruses, e.g. rubella, herpes, Newcastle disease virus, hepatitis virus, murine leukaemia viruses, leprosy bacilli, leishmania organisms, malaria parasites	Interference with immune induction by effects on T lymphocytes or macrophages
Trypanosomes Malaria parasites	Immunosuppressive effects, antigenic variation in successive generations so that antibody is ineffective
Schistosomes	Antigenic disguise by incorporating host antigens in cell wall
Neisseria gonorrhoea	Produces factor that breaks down IgA_1

importance as sites of attachment of microorganisms. Certain streptococci that are normal inhabitants of the mouth have been shown to adhere to epithelial cells of the cheek, whilst others preferentially attach to tooth surfaces. Specific attachment of various bacteria to different parts of the intestinal tract may account for the nature of the indigenous flora of the gut. It is suggested that the pathogenicity of *Salmonella typhii* and *Corynebacterium diptheriae* depends on their ability to attach to the intestinal or pharyngeal mucosa respectively and *Neisseria gonorrhoea* is believed to attach to epithelial cells of the genito urinary tract by means of its 'pili'. This organism at the same time appears to secrete an enzyme that breaks down secretory IgA_1, whilst IgA_2 is not affected.

Infection and inflammation

The innate immune mechanisms that protect the individual (mechanical barriers, antibacterial substances and phagocytosis) have been discussed in Chapter 2 and this discussion is concerned with the protective responses that form a second line of defence. The microorganism, having successfully avoided the innate immune mechanisms, starts to proliferate in the tissues and its toxic products trigger an inflammatory response. The response is initiated by the release of vasoactive amines, principally histamine and SRS–A from mast cells. The resulting increase in vascular permeability leads to an exudation of serum proteins including components of complement, antibodies, blood clotting factors and phagocytic cells. Phagocytic cells are attracted to the site of inflammation by chemotactic factors generated by interaction of components of the complement system with antibody. C3a and C5a components are the chemotaxins. Anaphylatoxins generated at the same time increase vascular permeability and further encourage exudation of fluid and cells at the site of inflammation.

Many types of microorganisms (e.g. staphylococci, streptococci) are effectively dealt with by the polymorphs and the intensity and duration of the inflammatory process depends on the degree of success with which the microorganism initially established itself. This in turn depending on the extent of the injury, the amount of associated tissue damage and the number and type of microorganisms introduced. A localized abscess may arise at the site of infection.

Some microorganisms (e.g. pneumococci) as mentioned above are able to resist phagocytosis and are not dealt with effectively until large amounts of antibody are made, sufficient to mop up the released capsular polysaccharide and then allow phagocytosis. If bacteria are not eliminated at the site of entry and continue to proliferate, they may pass via the lymphatics to the regional lymph nodes causing their enlargement (lymphadenitis). Other microorganisms (e.g. diphtheria, tetanus, cholera) produce exotoxins and are thus called **toxigenic** organisms. In this situation they can produce their damaging effects without migrating from their site of entry. Immunity in this situation requires the development of specific **antitoxins** (see below).

The types of infection described above are usually referred to as **acute infections** and contrast with protracted or **chronic infection** which is usually induced by microorganisms that are adapted to live within the cells of the host. Included amongst these are mycobacterial infections (e.g. tuberculosis, leprosy) brucella infections and virus infections. In these infections cell-mediated immunity plays a predominant part in the final elimination of the microorganism.

Immunity in bacterial infections

Antibody-mediated immunity

Antitoxins. Many microorganisms owe their pathogenic abilities to the production of **exotoxins**. Amongst diseases dependent on this type of mechanism are diphtheria, cholera, tetanus, gas gangrene and botulism.

Diphtheria toxin, for example, is a polypeptide chain with a molecular weight of about 62,000 daltons. The intact molecule is not active but requires the reduction of one disulphide bridge and hydrolysis of the peptide chain to release an active fragment. This is believed to occur at the membrane of host cells resulting in the entry of the toxic fragment into the cell where it interferes with protein synthesis. The cholera toxin owes its effects to its ability to bind to a specific glycolipid of the intestinal cell wall. A toxin constituent then passes through the cell wall, enters the cytoplasm and irreversibly 'switches on' the adenyl cyclase (the cyclic AMP-making enzyme). The 'activated' cell then proceeds to secrete fluid into the intestinal lumen resulting in massive fluid loss from the tissues.

Antibodies either acquired by immunization or previous infection, or given passively as antiserum, are able to **neutralize** bacterial toxins. To give protection, antibodies must either be present in sufficient quantity, as they would after administration of antiserum, or be produced faster than the toxin is produced by the microorganism. This would be likely to occur if the individual had previously been exposed to the organism or its products by natural

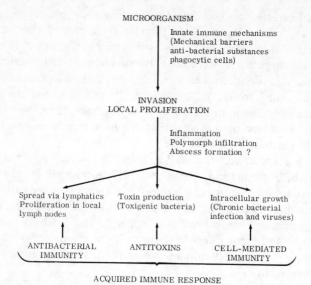

MICROORGANISM

Innate immune mechanisms
(Mechanical barriers
anti-bacterial substances
phagocytic cells)

INVASION
LOCAL PROLIFERATION

Inflammation
Polymorph infiltration
Abscess formation ?

Spread via lymphatics   Toxin production   Intracellular growth
Proliferation in local   (Toxigenic bacteria)   (Chronic bacterial
lymph nodes   infection and viruses)

ANTIBACTERIAL   ANTITOXINS   CELL-MEDIATED
IMMUNITY   IMMUNITY

ACQUIRED IMMUNE RESPONSE

Fig. 8.1 Scheme showing the progress of infection and the immunological defence mechanisms.

infection or artificial immunization. In such a situation the infected individual would be able to mount a rapid secondary immune response (p. 40). The previously exposed individual can be said to have an **immunological memory** of the toxin, having a population of cells ready and waiting to respond rapidly to the slightest whiff of the exotoxin. The infected individual with no 'immunological memory' may require to be given antibody prophylactically in order to tide him over the first stages of infection.

Bacterial toxins have been largely identified as enzymatic in nature and the antibody in some way is able to interfere with the ability of the enzyme to interact with its substrate. The antibody is not thought likely to interact with the active site of the enzyme but the nearer it reacts to this the more effective is its neutralizing power likely to be. The most probable explanation of the inhibitory effect of antibody is that it produces what is called 'steric hindrance', which simply means that it gets in the way and physically prevents the enzyme from coming in close apposition to its substrate (Fig. 8.2). To support this idea is the finding that antibody is much more effective against enzymes which have high molecular weight substrates than it is against those with low molecular weight substrates. Figure 8.2 shows how such a low molecular weight substrate can still come in contact with the active site of the enzyme even in the presence of antibody.

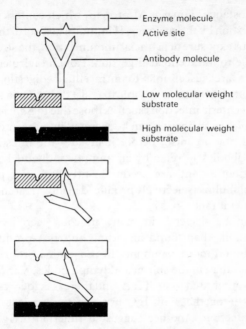

Fig. 8.2 Diagrammatic view of the possible 'steric hindrance' effect of antibody against an enzyme toxin. A low molecular weight substrate avoids the blocking effect of the antibody molecule. The closer the antibody is attached to the active site of the enzyme the more effective will be its blocking action.

Antibacterial immunity. In the case where a microorganism does not secrete exotoxins, the protection afforded by antibodies depends on the direct effect of antibodies attached to the surface of the microorganism. This can have a number of effects the most important of which is in encouraging phagocytosis by macrophages of the blood (monocytes) or the polymorphonuclear leucocytes. Phagocytic cells have receptors for a site on the Fc fragment of immunoglobulin G (particularly the human IgG 1 and IgG 3 subclasses) that is exposed after the immunoglobulin has combined with its antigen. There are also receptors for the C3b component of complement. This means that a bacterium coated with antibody and complement will adhere to a phagocytic cell and become susceptible to phagocytosis (see also p. 14). The phagocytic cell in many instances can then digest the microorganism by secreting into the phagocytic vacuole a variety of digestive enzymes carried in the intracellular lysosomes. However, some microorganisms such as the streptococci and *Mycobacterium tuberculosis* are able to resist intracellular digestion. The streptococcus carries, as part of its cell wall, a substance known as M protein, which confers the ability to resist digestion by the enzymes. If immunity exists to the M protein, by previous exposure or artificial immunization, the streptococcus is susceptible to intracellular digestion. Rough (avirulent) strains of salmonella are susceptible to intracellular digestion whilst the smooth (virulent) strains are able to resist digestion in some way. In the case of enteric infections such as those due to *Salmonella typhi* or *Vibrio cholerae*, antibodies can be secreted into the intestinal lumen and attack the organism before it invades the intestinal mucosa. These antibodies secreted by an immune individual are known as copro-antibodies and are predominantly IgA in type. The IgA immunoglobulin is selectively produced in intestinal and respiratory mucous membranes (p. 57).

IgA can be detected in many mucous secretions in higher concentrations than found in serum, and IgA-producing plasma cells are found more commonly in the lamina propria of mucous membranes than in the spleen and lymph nodes. Various functions have been attributed to such IgA, and there is evidence that it acts as an antitoxin together with IgG in protection against experimental cholera infection. Another suggested function of IgA is that by reacting with gut microorganisms it prevents their adherence to the gut wall. This is suggested by experiments in mice in which cholera organisms were prevented from adhering to the gut wall by the presence of IgA. A further function of IgA is suggested by work with IgA fractions of human colostrum, which bind to *E. coli* together with complement. The effect of this on the lipopolysaccharide of the bacterial cell wall is postulated to lead to the exposure of the underlying mucopeptide and enables the enzyme lysozyme (p. 11) to digest the mucopeptide layer with resulting lysis of the bacterium. Gram -ve organisms such as *E. coli* are normally resistant to the effects of lysozyme (Fig. 8.3). It should be noted that these effects have been shown by *in vitro* assays and may not reflect what occurs in the intact animal. Other effects of antibody reacting

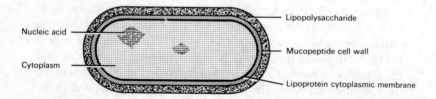

Fig. 8.3 Gram – ve bacillus showing lipopolysaccharide which protects mucopeptide cell wall from the effects of the mucolytic enzyme lysozyme. IgA + complement may attack the lipopolysaccharide and allow access of lysozyme to the cell wall.

with the surface of the microorganism are cell lysis, brought about by the activation of the complement system, and simple localization of the organism by agglutination or clumping.

It is even conceivable that antibody acts by coating growing bacteria so that their daughter cells, when formed, remain in a clump instead of dispersing. Attachment of bacteria to the host's red blood cells in the presence of antibody and complement is another way in which phagocytosis is encouraged. This phenomenon is known as **immune adherence** but as yet it is not clear exactly how the attachment to red cells takes place.

Apart from the clumping effect on the bacteria, agglutination seems to have little effect on the viability or respiratory activity of the organisms although it is conceivable that the bacteria at the centre of a large mass of clumped organisms would be limited in their metabolic activity simply by a lack of sufficient nutrient material. Recent work suggests that antibody can inhibit the uptake of iron by some bacteria and that its lack can inhibit their growth.

A possible protective role for IgE has been suggested by the finding of a similar distribution of this immunoglobulin to that found for IgA in the mucous secretions produced by local plasma cells. IgE is known to attach to the surface of mast cells and on combination with antigen, degranulation of the mast cell occurs with histamine release. These reactions in the allergic individual lead to hypersensitivity states (p. 96) but if occurring on a smaller scale in a localized area might be helpful in bringing about an inflammatory response with consequent elimination of a microorganism.

Acquired cellular immunity

Macrophage-dependent cellular immunity. The inter-relations of antibody-mediated immune mechanisms and acquired cellular immunity are not yet clearly defined. It is known, however, that macrophages from animals immune to tubercle bacilli are more actively phagocytic than those taken from a normal animal. The cells spread out more than unstimulated macrophages when cultured in a glass chamber, are more heavily endowed with mitochondria and lysosomes. The cellular immunity fades with time but can be recalled in an accelerated manner only by exposure to the original antigenic stimulus. Enhancement of cellular immunity has been reported with macrophages from brucella-infected animals; such cells restricted the intracellular growth of brucellae although the enhancement was dependent on the initial immunization with a living virulent strain of the organism. The same phenomenon has been found after *Liseria monocytogenes* infection in mice where macrophages isolated from the peritoneal cavity acquire an increased resistance to listeria and at the same time an increased intracellular resistance to tubercle bacilli and brucellae. This increased resistance is **non-specific** in the immunological sense in that the enhanced activity of the macrophage is directed not only at the species of organism responsible for the initial infection but also at other species (see Table 4.6).

The non-specific enhancement of macrophage activity, including their ability to kill microorganisms and spread themselves throughout the peritoneal cavity to mop up an infectious agent, appears to depend partly upon the transfer of an as yet undefined stimulus from lymphoid cells which have reacted immunologically to the initial injection of microorganisms. Thus the first part of the response depends on a specific immune reaction on the part of lymphoid cells to an agent such as *L. monocytogenes*; these cells proliferate and in turn activate the macrophages so that not only do they handle listeria more effectively but also other bacterial agents. This phenomenon can be shown quite clearly by transferring stimulated mouse lymphoid cells to an unstimulated recipient; the recipient's macrophages then assume these enhanced bactericidal and spreading properties. These points emphasize that cellular immunity, though non-specific in its expression, is specific in its elicitation and that the non-specific component is a property of the macrophage and the specific component dependent on the lymphocyte.

Immunity in virus infections
Antibody-mediated immunity
Bloodstream or surface protection. In virus infections the efficiency of antibody depends largely on whether the virus passes through the blood stream in order to reach its target organ. A well-known example of a virus which follows such a route is the **polio virus**; this crosses the intestinal wall, enters the blood stream and passes to the spinal cord and brain where it proliferates. Small amounts of antibody in the blood can **neutralize** the virus before it reaches its target cells in the nervous system. A number of other viruses behave in the same way and pass through the blood stream on their way to their target organ; examples are the viruses of measles, mumps, rubella and chickenpox. Disease caused by these viruses is characterized by a **prolonged** incubation period. In comparison, in another group of virus diseases with a **short** incubation period such as influenza and the common cold, the viruses do not pass through the blood stream, as their target organ is their site of entry to the

body, namely the respiratory mucous membranes. In this type of infection, even a high blood level of antibody will be relatively ineffective against these viruses in comparison with its effect on the blood-borne viruses. For this antibody to act on such respiratory viruses it must pass through the mucous membranes into the respiratory secretion. Examination of the antibody content of mucous secretion has shown that in contrast to the blood there is very little IgG antibody and often no IgM and it thus appears that the mucous membranes are not very permeable to antibodies of these classes. However, it has been found that the predominant immunoglobulin in these secretions is IgA manufactured by plasma cells in the lamina propria of the mucous membranes. IgA present in nasal secretions has been shown to be responsible for most of the neutralizing activity against common cold viruses. One conclusion which can be drawn from this is that conventional immunization methods designed to produce high blood levels of antibody are unlikely to be effective against viruses which attack the mucous membranes, and some effort is being directed at developing methods for stimulating local antibody production of IgA type in the mucous membranes themselves. An example of this is the intranasal administration of a live attenuated influenza virus which has been used extensively in the United States and the Soviet Union and is now available in Britain. The high degree of immunity provided by the oral polio vaccine seems likely in part to be due to locally produced antibody in the gut neutralizing the virus even before it reaches the blood stream. The presence of IgA antibody against polio virus has recently been demonstrated in the faeces, in duodenal fluid and in saliva. In contrast, after injection of inactivated virus vaccine no such antibodies could be found. The nasopharyngeal antibodies have been shown to persist for at least 300 days which is consistent with the long term protection which the oral vaccine affords. It is of some interest that the levels of IgA antipolio antibody were found to be lower in children who had their tonsils and adenoids removed. Furthermore primary vaccination in such children produced lower levels of these specific antibodies than in children who had not had their tonsils removed.

Persistence of virus and 'antigenic drift' One of the major differences between viral and bacterial immunity is that the former is usually of much longer duration and in many instances lifelong, e.g. in measles and mumps. An explanation of this may be that some virus remains within tissue cells and is protected from immune rejection. Occasionally some virus material is released and thus maintains a persisting level of immunity. The possibility exists that such virus antigen will combine with antibody resulting in the formation of **toxic complexes** with ensuing hypersensitivity of type 3 (p. 100). The existence of such a phenomenon could have considerable importance in the pathogenesis of some viral diseases.

In those virus infections in which repeated attacks occur, e.g. influenza and the common cold, fresh infection is due to different strains of the virus which are relatively insusceptible to the antibodies induced by previous infection by other strains. Evidence for a persisting immunity to virus comes from studies in the Faroe islands where successive measles epidemics were separated by intervals of 65 and 31 years. Only those who had not been previously infected developed the disease. Persistence of antibody can also be shown after virus and other infections, for example in Eskimos, 40 years after polio virus infection.

Influenza epidemics have occurred at 2 to 3 year intervals over the last 40 years and type B virus outbreaks tend to alternate with type A epidemics. Type A virus is responsible for pandemic influenza infections. Type C influenza virus rarely, if ever, gives rise to epidemics and no variants have been reported since it was first isolated in 1950. The main viral antigen responsible for inducing immunity is the haemagglutinin (HA). Sometimes called the 'V' antigen and is thought to be located on the spikes projecting from the viral envelope. Influenza viruses types A and B have different HA antigens and within these two types there are a number of distinct families with HA antigens which differ markedly from one another. Antigenic differences between HA antigens form the basis for classification of the viruses into families of the same type. Neuraminidase is also a surface antigen of influenza viruses and is responsible for the ability of the viruses to attach to tissue cells including red blood cells. This allows its laboratory detection in a haemagglutination test (see p. 183). In type A infection, the families A, A_0, A_1 and A_2 have appeared successively, and each in turn has dominated the epidemic history of influenza for periods of 10 to 15 years and is then displaced by later antigenic variants. It is believed that this 'antigen drift' from one virus family to another is one of progressive mutation, and that immunity against earlier strains becomes obsolete once further antigenic variants have appeared. The consequence of antigenic drift is that new strains do not react well with antisera against older strains, although older strains tend to react well with antibody against the new strain. Antigenic drift is probably due to selective pressures brought about by antibody that favours the emergence of mutants supressing surface antigens sufficiently different as to be unable to combine with existing antibody.

There is a danger that mutants responsible for 'antigen drift' may emerge and dominate as a result of widespread use of vaccination procedures directed against strains responsible for epidemics. In this situation such insusceptible mutants would be 'selected' from the virus population and replace the previously dominant strain.

The phenomenon of 'antigen drift' is not limited to influenza virus and the argument outlined above has been used for not instituting nationwide vaccination as a means of protecting cattle from foot and mouth disease virus. The same difficulties stand in the way of the development of common cold vaccines.

Cell-mediated immunity

Virus elimination and tissue damage. The humoral immune response is probably the predominant form of immunity responsible for protection from reinfection by viruses. For this reason immunization procedures aim at producing circulating or mucous membrane antibody. In the case of primary virus infections the position is not very clear but it seems likely to involve some form of cell-mediated immunity. It is known that children with congenital hypogammaglobulinaemia (p. 88) can recover from virus infections without producing any virus-neutralizing antibody. Although it is possible that these children are producing small amounts of neutralizing antibody sufficient to provide immunity, it is significant that the capacity to resist virus infection is associated with normal cell-mediated immune reactions. These subjects are able to develop normal delayed hypersensitivity reactions to bacterial and viral antigens and contact sensitivity to simple chemicals (p. 104). In patients with Swiss-type agammaglobulinaemia (p. 90), who have an additional cell-mediated immune deficiency, susceptibility to virus infection is very great and death often follows the development of severe generalized vaccinia after routine inoculation of live smallpox vaccine.

A laboratory model is available that has enabled the detailed study of the role of cell-mediated immunity in virus infection. Adult mice infected with lymphocytic choriomeningitis virus (LCM virus), which itself is not damaging to cells (non-cytopathic), develop clinical signs (e.g. meningitis) with the onset of an immune response to the virus. If this response is prevented by means of immunosuppressive agents (e.g. anti-lymphocyte serum, cytotoxic drugs, irradiation or thymectomy) then the disease does not develop. If an infected animal treated in this way is then given

spleen cells from an untreated virus infected animal, the pathological changes characteristic of the disease develop in the recipient.
These changes are likely to be brought about by a cytotoxic factor
(p. 75) released from the transferred spleen cells interacting with
infected cells of the recipient. The consequences of this immune
response can thus be seen to be twofold: (1) virus infected cells are
destroyed by stimulated spleen cells with the likely elimination of
the virus; (2) host cells are themselves damaged and this is
responsible for the pathological manifestations of the disease.
Whether or not the pathological changes in any human virus
infections depend on mechanisms of this type is not clear at present.
However, some *in vitro* experiments in which cells infected with
measles or mumps virus are destroyed by incubation with spleen
cells of a virus-immunized animal suggest that such phenomena
may take place in the disease state itself. Much additional work will
be required before the picture becomes clear.

Further evidence that cell-mediated immune reactions are
involved in resistance to viruses comes from the finding that, just as
in the case of intracellular bacterial agents such as tubercle bacilli
and brucellae, cell-mediated reactions of the delayed hypersensitivity type (p. 103) can be demonstrated after many types of
virus infection. The best known example of this is the reaction soon
after revaccination with vaccinia virus where there is an accelerated
reaction (compared to primary vaccination) reaching its maximum
at 72 hours with a minimum of tissue damage and a rapid
elimination of the infective agent.

Babies with congenital rubella infection have been shown to
excrete virus for periods up to 18 months of age. Such infants can be
shown to possess high levels of IgM anti-rubella antibody, which
indicates that they have not developed neonatal tolerance (p. 69) to
the virus. Their cell-mediated immune mechanisms seem, however, to be defective due to a direct effect of the virus on
lymphocytes. Lymphocytes taken from such an infant do not
respond normally to the plant mitogen PHA (p. 73) and normal
leucocytes infected *in vitro* with the virus can be shown to become
defective in the same way. **Depression of lymphocyte reactivity**
has been associated with a number of virus infections, e.g. rubella,
herpes, Newcastle disease virus (causing fowl pest) and hepatitis
virus. Certain viruses are able to **replicate** in **macrophages** (e.g.
arboviruses, murine hepatitis virus, lactate dehydrogenase virus and
herpes simplex virus) and others do so in **lymphocytes** (e.g.
lymphocytic choriomeningitis virus, leukaemia viruses and Epstein-
Barr virus).

The effects on the activity of the immune system brought about by viral infection have been mainly studied with murine leukaemia viruses. Infection of mice with these viruses usually results in depression of the activity of the immune system affecting both humoral and cell-mediated immunity. In some instances (e.g. Friend virus infection) there is selective depression of a particular class of immunoglobulin (IgG) suggesting an effect on particular populations of lymphocytes. Graft rejection was found to be profoundly depressed in animals infected with gross leukaemia virus.

The mechanisms underlying these effects are not clear. Amongst the proposed mechanisms are: virus induced changes in the **uptake** and processing of antigens; **destruction** of cells of the immune systems; antigenic **competition** by the virus preventing the host response to other antigens.

The clinical implications include persistence of virus in the absence of a protective immune response; the development of immune complex disease (p. 101); potentiation of tumour growth as a result of depressed immunological capacity and thus of immune surveillance mechanisms (p. 167).

Recent studies have indicated that the lesions associated with virus infections cannot be explained simply by the cytopathic effects of the virus on cells. The immune response of the host to the viral antigen appears to play a role in producing tissue damage due to the immune complexes (see p. 101), formed by virus and antibody.

Another way in which a virus can initiate destruction of host cells is by virus induced changes in the surface antigens of the host cell. The altered surface antigen stimulates an immune response with subsequent destruction of the cell by antibody and complement and possible concomitant release of pharmacologically active mediators of inflammation (p. 95). Such a phenomenon is not necessarily detrimental only to the host cells as these are virus infected cells and their elimination would lead also to destruction of the virus. In conclusion it can be seen that the outcome of a virus infection is the result of the **interplay** between **protective** and **hypersensitivity** mechanisms the balance usually settling in favour of protection. Figure 8.4 is an attempt to summarize these complex interrelationships.

Interferon. A quite distinct type of resistance mechanism in virus infection is the production by the infected host cells of a substance known as 'interferon'. This material interferes with the synthesis of

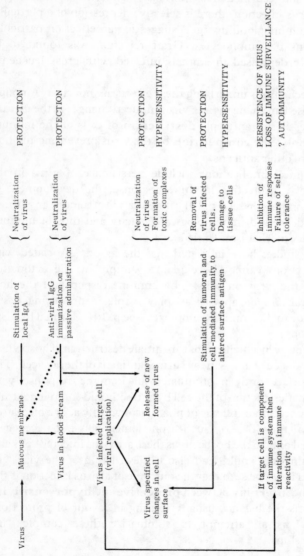

Fig. 8.4 Schematic view of virus infection and immune response, indicating some possible consequences.

new virus by tissue cells of the host. Interferon, unlike antibody, is not specific for the virus which may have induced its formation but is able to interfere with other quite different species of virus. Interferon probably plays a very important role in eliminating virus in non-immune individuals and the rise in level of interferon appears to coincide with the phase of virus elimination whilst circulating antibody levels are found to rise subsequent to this.

Susceptibility to virus disease and immune response genes

In Chapter 4 consideration has been given to the genetic control of the immune response by a specific group of genes called **Ir genes**. These have been shown to be closely related to those genes controlling the major antigenic determinants of graft rejection (MHC genes). The possibility that a gene product closely associated with the MHC genes is involved in co-operation between T and B lymphocytes leading to an immune response is noted on p. 84. This phenomenon is of interest in view of the known relationship between histocompatibility antigens (determined by the MHC gene complex) and susceptibility to certain virus-induced leukaemias in mice. The susceptibility of mice to lymphocytic-choriomeningitis virus (p. 127) may also be determined in this way. With increased knowledge of the gene complex controlling histocompatibility antigens and various functions of lymphocytes associated with the immune response, it should be possible in the next few years to elucidate some of the factors that determine susceptibility to virus diseases.

Immunity to protozoa and helminths

The life cycles of organisms in this category are complicated and the immune response to be effective has to interrupt the cycle at a stage when the parasite is accessible to the immune processes.

Protozoa. Malaria infections are initiated by sporozoites which transform into exoerythrocytic schizonts in the liver, and at this stage there is recognizable immunity. The schizonts rupture and discharge their merozoites into the peripheral circulation where they invade erythrocytes. Antibodies are readily detectable in the serum and increase until the crisis 7 to 10 days later and then slowly decline. Because these antibodies are able to get access to the parasite only during a relatively short period of its life cycle, immunity is incomplete and the host usually fails to eliminate the parasite completely.

This state in which the organisms persist in small numbers in the tissues in the presence of an immune reaction is called **premunition** by parasitologists.

The IgG class of immunoglobulin is the major antibody class involved in acquired resistance to malaria and there is a considerable rise in the levels of, and rate of synthesis of, the IgG. However, if serum from an infected individual is incubated with parasitized erythrocytes, only a small quantity of the IgG antibody is absorbed. The major part of the IgG probably represents antibody to soluble malarial antigens, and seems unlikely to play a role in protection except perhaps when it is directed against toxic malarial products. Parasitic growth within erythrocytes is unaffected by the presence of immune serum in the culture medium, but invasion of new red cells by merozoites and subsequent parasite multiplication is inhibited. IgG antibodies can bind to Fc receptors on macrophages (p. 63) and it seems likely that phagocytosis of antibody coated merozoites is an important mechanism of acquired immunity. There is evidence that antibody may act on mature intraerythrocytic forms of the parasite possibly due to expression of parasite antigen on the surface of the red cells that render the red cells susceptible to attack by antibody.

Considerable experimental evidence exists showing that malarial infection is associated with **immunosuppression** and that the extent of this parallels the degree of parasitaemia. It is not clear whether this has an effect on the immune response to the parasite itself, but depressed responsiveness of T lymphocytes to PHA (p. 73) and B lymphocytes to bacterial lipopolysaccharide can readily be demonstrated, as can diminished antibody responses to certain antigens. Further work will show the relative importance of cell-mediated and humoral immunity in malaria infections but at the moment humoral immunity appears to be the predominant protective mechanism.

The efficacy of the immune mechanisms against trypanosomes is complicated by the fact that the parasites can change their surface antigenic constitution from one generation to the next. The number of variants which can be produced by a single strain is at least 20. It is not yet clear how the organism controls the generation of the variants but variation is thought to arise by selection of mutants from a heterogeneous population of parasites.

This complication means that the immune response has great difficulty in keeping up with the antigenic changes in the parasite, and in the case of the trypanosomes responsible for African sleeping sickness the parasite does not induce an effective immunity, the infected subject developing a progressive infection with invasion of the central nervous system leading to death. Trypanosomiasis is associated with high levels of IgM immunoglobulins in both the blood and CSF. It is not certain if this is due to the repeated new antigenic stimuli resulting from changes in the organism or if the parasite in some way influences directly the cells of the immune system. Increased immunoglobulin production is a common finding in protozoal infections and often affects all classes of immunoglobulins. Because usually less than 5 per cent of the total immunoglobulin appears to react specifically with the inducing parasite it is probable that protozoa stimulate the lymphoid cells in a non-specific way to overproduce immunoglobulins.

Helminths. Helminths like protozoa go through a complex life cycle and protective immune mechanisms appear to act only at an early stage in the cycle. The main stimulus appears to be due to antigens derived from the adult worm and the immunity derived from this acts on new parasites entering the body. A noteworthy feature of these infections is the appearance of IgE (reaginic) antibodies (p. 96) with pulonary eosinophilia, and it seems likely that immediate ate hypersensitivity reactions of the anaphylactic type (type 1) are involved in the pathogenesis of helminth infection. In schistosomiasis mansoni infections the pathogenesis appears to be largely due to an **inflammatory granulomatous reaction** around the **schistosome eggs** trapped in the host tissues with a periovular area of necrosis surrounded by inflammatory cells, including many eosinophils. The most severe lesions occur during early infection. Mice in experimental schistosomiasis infections reject 70 to 80 per cent of new infections 12 weeks after their first infection. In baboons a significant reduction, in the damage done by the parasite to the host organs, was found in pre-immunized animals. The experimental findings suggest a gradual waning of egg hypersensitivity but the mechanism is not understood. The tissues commonly affected are the liver, which shows chronic portal inflammation, the lungs, the kidneys and the spleen. The renal and splenic lesions are not directly related to the presence of worms or eggs, but may in part be due to immune complexes between worm antigens and antibody. In schistosomiasis haematobium the urinary tract is the primary target and calcification of the bladeer can occur in advanced cases. It has been suggested that the activation of pharmacological mediators by the IgE–antigen interaction may be a valuable defence mechanism. The associated increase in vascular permeability would be likely to allow access to the site of infection of immunocompetent cells, antibody and complement. Migration of larvae into the lungs is sometimes associated with eosinophil infiltration and pneumonia which can be fatal.

Another role for IgE in protection against worm infestation is its ability to adhere to macrophages. This brings about attachment of the parasite to macrophages, which may lead to the death of the parasite. This possibility is suggested by experiments with worms in schistosomal infections in which *in vitro* killing of the worms by macrophages was greatly accelerated when IgE antibody to the worm was present. These worms are believed to be able to protect themselves from host antibody by **incorporating host tissue antigens** in their cell wall. When worms are transferred from mice to monkeys that are immunized against mouse red blood cells, the worms are killed by an antibody-mediated reaction directed at the surface of the parasite. The host antigens acquired by the worms appear to be A, B and H blood group substances (p. 155) and possibly the Lewis antigen.

Saprophytic fungi and respiratory disease

Allergic alveolitis and anaphylaxis. A few examples of pulmonary hypersensitivity to inhaled fungal antigens have been reported in the last few years. The existence of a state of immunity has been confirmed by the finding of precipitating antibodies in the serum. The first of these disorders to be recognized was **farmers' lung** disease in which precipitating antibodies could be demonstrated against antigens derived from mouldy hay. The antigen has since been found to be *Microspora faeni*. Subsequently work in Edinburgh has demonstrated precipitins against *Aspergillus clavatus* in **maltworkers** exposed to high concentrations of *A. clavatus* spores from contaminated barley. Antibodies against *Coniosporum corticale* have been found in the serum of maple bark strippers.

It is likely that following exposure to high concentrations of any of a variety of fungal spores individuals would produce precipitating antibodies and thus this form of pulmonary hypersensitivity may be more widespread than has so far been identified. The hypersensitivity reaction induced by the presence of precipitating antibodies would be of the toxic-complex (type 3) form inducing a diffuse pulmonary interstitial pneumonitis which has been termed allergic alveolitis. Some of the antigens responsible for this form of hypersensitivity can also provoke in susceptible individuals the anaphylactic (type 1) response exemplified by pulmonary asthma. If growth of the fungus should occur in the lungs, as in the case of *Aspergillus fumigatus*, the metabolic products of the organism will cause further immunization and increase in precipitating antibodies

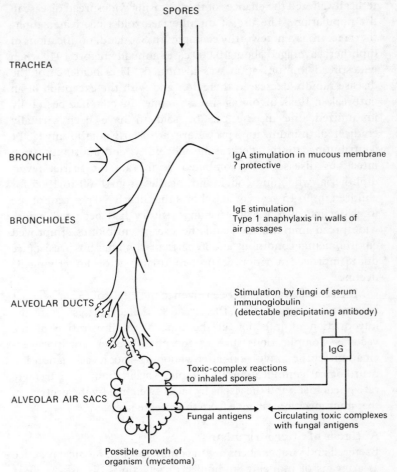

Fig. 8.5 Scheme showing some of the possible consequences that may result from the inhalation of fungal spores.

with the development of an accumulation of inflammatory cells at the site of infection. Figure 8.5 illustrates some of the possible consequences of a fungal respiratory infection.

Common vaccination procedures

Efficacy and hazards. It is generally accepted that one effective way of controlling the spread of infectious disease is by immunization with antigens derived from the appropriate organism. The isolation and bulk preparation of the particular antigens which confer protective immunity is a major difficulty, but success in this field with a number of potentially dangerous microorganisms has radically altered the chances of them causing widespread disease in the population. The use of diphtheria toxoid (inactivated diphtheria toxin) is a noteworthy example. In Scotland, notifications of diphtheria averaged about 10,000 cases annually before 1940 when widespread immunization was instituted. The incidence of the disease rapidly decreased thereafter and with the exception of an outbreak in 1968, involving six cases none of whom had been fully immunized, the disease can be said to have been virtually eradicated. Immunization procedures are clearly not the only factor contributing to the decreasing morbidity and mortality from infectious disease. The combined death rate for scarlet fever, diphtheria, whooping cough and measles from 1860 to 1965 for children up to 15 years of age shows that nearly 90 per cent of the total decline over the intervening century had occurred before widespread immunization and the use of antibiotics. Improved environmental conditions and in particular, higher host-resistance due to improved nutrition, are probably major factors underlying the decline.

Much consideration has been given to the safety of vaccines and it is generally agreed that the greatest danger arises from the introduction of infection at the time of administration of the vaccine. Complications such as encephalitis after smallpox vaccination, febrile convulsions after whooping-cough vaccination and neurological complication after rabies vaccination are extremely rare phenomena and the risk is by far outweighed by the protection that immunization can give from the disease itself.

Antigens of microorganisms

Bacterial and viral antigens are in common use in medical practice as a means of inducing immunity to infectious diseases such as smallpox, diphtheria, measles, poliomyelitis, typhoid fever and many others. There are four main types of antigen preparations or **vaccines.**

1. **Toxoids** are the soluble exotoxins of bacteria such as diphtheria and tetanus bacilli, which have been modified and rendered less toxic by the addition of formalin or gentle heating. They are administered either in solution or precipitated on alum. Many years of useful immunity can be achieved by these procedures.

2. **Killed vaccines** are cultured organisms killed by heat, usually 60°C for 1 hour, ultraviolet irradiation or chemicals such as phenol, alcohol or formalin. Protection against whooping cough, poliomyelitis and perhaps cholera can be achieved in this way.

3. **Antigens isolated from infectious agents,** for example the capsular polysaccharide of the pneumococci. A diffusable factor of *B. anthracis* and a cell wall preparation of haemolytic streptococci have been shown to induce immunity, but such preparations are not in general use in medical practice.

4. **Attenuated living vaccines** are made from strains of organisms that have lost their virulence by growth in culture (e.g. Pasteur's chicken cholera vaccine, p. 2) or in animals when the conditions are not favourable for the growth and proliferation of the virulent strain. Strains emerge which, whilst not able to produce disease, can induce immunity; such strains are known as **attenuated** organisms. The BCG vaccine (Bacille Calmette-Guérin) is the outstanding example of this type of vaccine, providing protection against tuberculosis in man. The oral administration of a strain of poliomyelitis virus induces a powerful immunity without producing the disease. The virus spreads from one individual to another and so is able to produce immunity in a community. An attenuated strain of yellow fever virus has been developed, obtained from the original virulent material by prolonged cultivation in tissue culture. Attenuated strains of measles virus are also used, and it seems likely that rubella virus vaccination will soon reduce the hazard of congenital abnormalities developing in the infants of mothers infected with the virus.

In veterinary medicine successful vaccines have been produced against canine distemper, canine hepatitis and Newcastle disease (fowl pest) of chickens.

Routine procedures

The determining factors in the selection of immunization procedures for a particular population must depend on local environmental conditions and epidemiological considerations. In Britain, a child is immunized during its first year of life with a vaccine containing diphtheria and tetanus toxoids in combination with a killed suspension of whooping-cough (*Bordetella pertussis*) organisms. This is known as **triple vaccine** and its efficacy as an immunizing agent is in part due to the adjuvant effect of the pertussis component. This procedure is repeated on two further occasions and at the same time oral polio vaccine is usually given. Vaccination against smallpox is achieved by giving one dose of the vaccinia vaccine during the second year when the chances of developing complications appear to be much decreased. Primary vaccination is not advised after early childhood. The risk of serious complications in early childhood is very small but nevertheless

Table 8.2 A schedule of vaccination and immunization procedures. After Department of Health and Social Security (1969).

Age	Prophylactic	Interval	Notes
During the first year of life	Diph/Tet/Pert and oral Polio vaccine. (First dose)		The earliest age at which the first dose should be given is 3 months, but a better general immunological response can be expected if the first dose is delayed to 6 months of age
	Diph/Tet/Pert and oral Polio vaccine. (Second dose)	Preferably after an interval of 6 to 8 weeks	
	Diph/Tet/Pert and oral Polio vaccine. (Third dose)	Preferably after an interval of 6 months	
During the second year of life	Measles vaccination Smallpox vaccination (see text)	An interval of 3 to 4 weeks should be allowed to elapse between giving two live vaccines or Diph/Tet/Pert and a live vaccine, other than oral polio	While the second year is recommended for vaccination against smallpox in special circumstances it may be carried out during the first year (see text)
At 5 years of age or school entry	Diph/Tet and oral Polio vaccine or Diph/Tet/Polio vaccine Smallpox revaccination		With the exception of smallpox revaccination these may be given, if desired at 3 years of age to children entering nursery schools, attending day nurseries or living in children's homes
Between ages 10 and 13 For tuberculin-negative children	BCG vaccine		
Between 11 and 13 (Girls only)	Rabella vaccine		
Between 15 and 19 years of age or on leaving school	Polio vaccine (oral or inactivated). Tetanus toxoid. Smallpox revaccination		

considered to be out of proportion to the risk of being infected with the disease. Thus smallpox vaccination need no longer be recommended as a routine procedure in early childhood. Booster doses of all these vaccines are usually given at 5 years of age and tetanus, polio and smallpox again between the ages of 15 and 19. Table 8.2 shows the recommended schedules of the Department of Health and Social Security.

In the U.S.A. the official recommendation for childhood immunization comprises the three primary doses of Diph/Tet/Pert vaccine and oral Polio vaccine at intervals of 4 to 6 weeks, beginning at the age of 2 to 3 months. A booster is given 1 year after completion of the primary course.

Live vaccines should not be given to persons whose ability to respond to infection is reduced, as for example after radiotherapy, immunosuppressive drugs, steroids or in patients with immune-deficiency states. If a subject has had a local or general reaction to a vaccine, there is a risk of even more marked reactions to the next dose.

FURTHER READING

Bulletin of the World Health Organization (1972) Virus-associated immuno-pathology: animal models and implications for human disease. *Bull. Wld Hlth Org.*, 47, 257.

Bulletin of the World Health Organization (1974) Immunology of schistosomiasis. *Bull. Wld Hlth Org.*, 51, 553.

Collee, J. G. (1976) *Applied Medical Microbiology*. Oxford: Blackwell.

Evans, D. G. (1969) Immunization against infectious diseases. *Br. med. Bull.*, 25, No. 2.

Gell, P. G. H., Coombs, R. R. A. & Lachmann, P. J. (Eds.) (1975) *Clinical Aspects of Immunology*. 3rd edition. Oxford: Blackwell.

Hobson, D. (1967) Immunization against respiratory virus infection. In *Modern Trends in Immunology*, 2, p. 53, ed. Cruickshank, R. & Weir, D. M. London: Butterworth.

Notkins, A. L. & Koprowski, H. (1973) How the immune response to a virus can cause disease. *Scientific American*, 228, 22.

World Health Organization (1975) Developments in malaria immunology. *Wld Hlth Org.*, Technical report series no. 579.

Youmans, G. P., Paterson, P. Y. & Somers, H. M. (Eds.) (1975) *The Biological and Clinical Basis of Infectious Diseases*. Philadelphia: Saunders.

9

Autoimmunity

A fundamental characteristic of an animal's immune system is that it does not under normal circumstances react against its own body constituents. There exists a mechanism which enables the cells of the immune system to recognize what is 'foreign' and what is 'self'. Attempts to explain the absence of reactions against self go back to the early days of immunology when Paul Ehrlich enunciated his well known doctrine of 'horror autotoxicus'. Ehrlich and Morgenroth in 1900, after immunizing a goat with red blood cells of other goats, found that although the animal readily made antibodies against the red cells of other goats these antibodies failed to react with the animal's own red cells. It was thus clear that in some way the immunological response to self antigens was prevented. So powerful was the influence of Paul Ehrlich that it seemed inconceivable that in any circumstances the rule could be broken so that an immunological reaction against self could develop. The view continued to be held despite clinical evidence indicating that diseases existed in which the patient was apparently destroying his own cells.

The main reason that observations of this type failed to achieve the recognition they deserved was the absence of serological techniques capable of demonstrating convincingly the existence of antibodies able to react with tissue cells or of the presence of such antibodies actually attached to cells. It was not until 1945 that immunologists were provided with this vital tool, when Coombs, Mourant and Race described a technique which detected the presence of antibody globulin on red blood cells by the simple expedient of adding an antiserum against human globulin which, after reacting with the globulin coating the cells, linked the cells together and agglutinated them. This method was particularly valuable for showing antibody globulin adsorbed to cells which was in itself unable to agglutinate the cells. This technique is commonly known as the 'Coombs' or 'antiglobulin' test (p. 182). The development of the antiglobulin techniques led to the use of antiglobulin sera in a variety of different ways many of which involved complicated technical operations but which essentially were based on the original antiglobulin method. Amongst the most important of the developments of the method is the fluorescent antibody technique in which one of the most commonly used procedures is to label an antiglobulin serum with a fluorescent marker (fluorescein isothiocyanate) so that the reaction of the labelled antiglobulin with, for example, globulin-coated cells can be visualized under UV light microscopy. Under these conditions the sites of attachment of the fluorescein-labelled antiglobulin show up as bright apple-green fluorescent areas (p. 186).

The recognition of autoimmune disease

These methods allowed a breakthrough in the recognition of a variety of human and animal diseases in which antibodies could be convincingly demonstrated in serum capable of reacting with a number of different antigens of the individual's own tissues.

The first of these was the demonstration that in some types of haemolytic anaemia in man the red blood cells were coated with antibody globulin. This was soon followed by the finding of an autoantibody serum factor in the blood of patients with a severe connective tissue disease called systemic lupus erythematosus (SLE). This factor appeared to be antibody against the nuclei of tissue cells and was called by the author and his colleagues antinuclear factor (ANF). At the same time workers interested in diseases of the thyroid gland demonstrated the presence of an antibody to thyroglobulin in patients with a particular form of interstitial thyroiditis known as Hashimoto's disease.

The first recognizable clinical description of acquired haemolytic anaemia was given in 1898 in France, and in 1908 haemolytic activity against red cells was found in the serum of patients in whom intense haemolysis was taking place *in vivo*. These early observations were neglected until 30 years later when Damashek and Schwartz again reported haemolysins in patients suffering from haemolytic anaemia, and with the introduction of the Coombs test in 1945 the immunological basis of the disease was put on a firm foundation.

The effect on immunological theory

Associated with the accumulating evidence on the autoimmune nature of the haemolysins in acute haemolytic anaemia, there arose the need to consider the meaning of foreignness and self-recognition and the mechanisms underlying the ability of the body to differentiate between 'self' and 'non-self'. A solution to the problem this created in immunological theory was offered by Burnet and Fenner in 1949. At that time antibody production was envisaged in terms of the antigen acting as a template for modifying the globulin molecules to a form which was complementary to that of antigen (p. 68). It was considered that antigen might act either on the already formed protein chain and bring about a reconfiguration of the chain, or that the antigen induced a chemical rearrangement of the globulin molecule as it was formed. Burnet and Fenner, whilst accepting this direct template theory, included the notion of 'self-markers' attached to body components by which antibody-forming cells were able to recognize them, thus rendering them immunologically inert. They also predicted that an equivalent tolerance to foreign antigens should be demonstrable if these had been introduced at an appropriate stage in embryonic life, while the animal's immune system was in the process of learning to recognize the 'self-markers' of its own tissues. This prediction was later confirmed experimentally by Medawar and his colleagues who showed that if neonatal mice were injected with transplantation antigen from another strain of mice, they would later be able to accept skin grafts which an animal not injected neonatally would rapidly reject.

Burnet soon followed his 'self-marker' theory by his rather more plausible '**clonal selection**' theory. This allowed the antigen no part in impressing a pattern on the antibody-producing cells. The capacity to produce a given antibody was regarded as a genetically determined quality of certain clones or families of mesenchymal cells, the function of the antigen being to stimulate cells of these clones to proliferation and antibody production. The theory postulated that in the early stages of embryonic development, mutation of cells led to a variety of **random** arrangements in the globulin molecules so that a very large number of clones were generated which could correspond to potential antigenic determinants (p. 71). To explain the inability of the antibody-forming system to react with self, Burnet proposed that the immature cells could be destroyed if they came across the antigens with which they could react at this early stage. Whenever the antigenic determinants were freely present in the body and accessible to the corresponding immunologically competent cells, such destructive contacts would be inevitable. Tolerance would result from the elimination or inhibition of all cell clones which had the ability to react with antigenic determinants present in the body. After birth when foreign antigen entered the tissues antibody to it would be produced by specific stimulation of those cells in clones preadapted to react with the corresponding antigenic determinants. On the basis of this theory Burnet accounted for the development of autoimmune disease as a failure of the destruction of the self-reactive population of antibody-forming cells (see also p. 65).

Possible mechanisms involved in the development of autoimmunity

The question now arises of how the normal controlling mechanism fails with the resulting inability to maintain self-recognition manifested by immune reactions against self.

Table 9.1 Mechanisms of autoantibody formation

---

1. **Evasion** of normal tolerance to 'self' antigens
   - (a) Hidden antigens
   - (b) Altered antigens –
     chemicals, drugs,
     infectious agents

2. **Breakdown** of tolerance mechanism
   - (a) Agents affecting antibody forming cells –
     chemicals, drugs,
     infectious agents
   - (b) Genetically determined lack of efficiency of tolerance control mechanisms (e.g. by suppressor T cells)

3. **Stimulation** of pre-existing B cell population capable of self-reactivity
   - (a) Infectious agents and adjuvants (? effects on suppressor T cells)

There are three main ways (Table 9.1) in which this tolerance-maintaining mechanism could conceivably be overcome. The first involves evasion or circumvention of a normally functioning mechanism and the second failure of the mechanism itself. The third possible mechanism involves the stimulation of a pre-existing quiescent self-reactive B lymphocyte population.

In the first category evasion may occur in two possible ways: (1) because a particular body antigen is not accessible to the cells of the immune system as the antigen is hidden within a cell or tissue – these antigens are known as **sequestered** antigens; (2) because a tissue antigen is **altered** in some way by a chemical agent, a drug or an infectious agent.

Sequestered antigens. Hidden or sequestered antigens do seem to exist and the best examples of these are sperm antigens and lens antigen of the eye. Sperm can be shown to acquire an antigen during maturation which is absent from the immature germinal cells and antibodies can be induced in the guinea-pig by immunizing with autologous sperm showing that the immune system fails to recognize the sperm as part of self. Orchitis can be induced by combining the sperm with an adjuvant which gives a boost to the immune response and at the same time in some way allows the stimulated lymphoid cells and antibody to gain access to the sperm-forming tissues. Orchitis in man is a rare complication of mumps infection in which it is assumed that the virus damages the basement membrane barrier of the seminiferous tubules and the cells of the immune system are thus allowed entry and initiate an immune response.

In the case of the lens it can be shown that if a rabbit is injected with bovine lens material, it develops antibodies which react with its own lens *in vitro*. Occasionally the surgical extraction of a lens for cataract is succeeded by inflammatory changes in retained lens substance sometimes affecting the other unoperated lens, and the same phenomenon can be induced experimentally in animals.

Interpretation of observations of this type is fraught with complications and can be regarded at present only as speculative evidence to support the concept of sequestered antigens as an initiating factor in autoimmune disease.

Altered antigens. Evidence in support of the second proposed way in which normal tolerance mechanisms are circumvented is more concrete. Experimental studies of tolerance evasion by altered antigens have been carried out with purified proteins, conjugates of hapten and protein, and with cellular antigens. Some of the most definitive work is that carried out in America by Weigle who showed that rabbits made tolerant to bovine serum albumen (BSA) and then immunized with the cross-reacting antigen human serum albumen (HSA) eventually made antibodies which could react with BSA. The same result was obtained with chemically modified BSA. A closer approximation to autoimmune disease is provided by experiments using thyroglobulin in rabbits; not only are anti-rabbit thyroglobulin antibodies induced by injection of altered thyroglobulin but inflammatory lesions are also found in their thyroid glands.

Shared antigens. There has been considerable interest in the last few years in the role of microorganisms as a source of cross-reacting antigens sharing antigenic determinants with tissue components.

The ability of viruses to bring about alterations of cell membranes has been suggested by studies on the effect of herpes and rabies viruses on tissue culture cells. New cell surface antigens (neoantigens) which appear to act as transplantation antigens, have been found in mouse cells infected with herpes and also with polyoma viruses.

There is an antigen in human colon extractable even from sterile foetal human colon, which is similar to a polysaccharide antigen present in *E. coli* 014. It is conceivable that the inflammatory condition of the colon known as ulcerative colitis, in which anticolon antibodies are found, is due to an immune reaction initiated by the cross-reacting bacterial antigen. Similarly the Group A streptococci, which are closely associated with rheumatic fever, have an antigen in common with a human heart antigen. Heart lesions are a common finding in rheumatic fever and anti-heart antibody is found in just over 50 per cent of patients with the condition.

Nephritogenic strains of Type 12 Group A streptococci carry surface antigens similar to those found in human glomeruli and infection by these organisms has been associated with the development of acute nephritis.

Drugs as haptens. Drugs can act as haptens (p. 21) which bind to tissue proteins. The resulting complex may be antigenic and result in an immune reaction which damages cells coated with the drug. An example of this is a metabolic breakdown product of the drug α-methyldopa (used in the treatment of hypertension). The immune response generated by these drug-altered cells can then result in haemolysis of the affected cells and α-methyldopa is thought to have the effect of altering or exposing normally hidden red cell antigens. The antibody which results has been found to combine with Rhesus antigens present on the surface of the patient's own normal erythrocytes. One hypothesis is that the α-methyldopa is incorporated into the Rhesus antigen when the red cell is being made and the change this induces prevents the antigen being recognized as self. (See also discussion of the effects of the drug Sedormid, p. 100.)

Disturbed immunological mechanisms. The second main category of mechanisms by means of which autoimmune reactions may develop (Table 9.1) are those due to alteration in the cellular processes on which maintenance of normal tolerance depends. One way in which this might occur is by the direct effect of a chemical, a drug or an infectious agent on the lymphoid tissues. Alternatively, it is conceivable that the loss of normal tolerance control might be due to an inherited defect or lack of efficiency in the lymphoid cell population. The existence of a T lymphocyte population (Suppressor T cells) that controls B lymphocyte activity has been noted on page 64. Suppressor T cells may prevent development of autoimmunity in the normal animal by recognizing any idiotypic determinants (p. 65) of anti-self immunoglobulins expressed on the B cell surface. It is conceivable that a defect (inherited or induced) of such suppressor T cells might allow B cells of this type to escape and produce anti-self immunoglobulin.

There is much speculation amongst immunologists and clinicians on the role of infectious agents acting **directly** on the lymphoid tissues as a cause of autoimmune disease. This stems from the experimental evidence on the induction of autoimmune disease using tissue antigens combined with Freund's complete adjuvant. This water-in-oil emulsion owes its powerful stimulating effect on the lymphoid tissues, to killed mycobacteria which are incorporated in the oil. Without the mycobacterial component, tissue antigens are much less effective in disturbing the tolerance mechanisms. Rabbits injected with *Mycobacterium tuberculosis* alone, have been shown to develop autoantibodies against a wide range of autologous tissues. The same phenomenon is found in a number of chronic infections in the human such as syphilis, actinomycosis and chronic tuberculosis. Infection with *Mycoplasma pneumoniae*, responsible for a disease known as primary atypical pneumonia, is associated with the development of IgM agglutinins in the patient's serum, which in the cold will react with the patient's own red cells.

A leukaemia virus has in the last few years been found in a strain of mice (New Zealand Black or NZB mice) characterized by the early development of autoimmune disease including autoimmune haemolytic anaemia and immune complex nephritis. The virus has been found in many body tissues and in the blood and can be seen in lymphoid organs, attached to the surface of lymphocytes. Similar virus particles have been found in embryos of the NZB strain, suggesting that it is passed through the placenta or is associated with the germ cells. The association of the virus with lymphocyte membranes has attracted the attention of immunologists and there has been speculation that the presence of the virus might interfere with normal lymphocyte reactivity to antigens. It is known (p. 60) that antigens can react with the lymphocyte surface and that this is probably one stimulus to immune transformation of these cells. The virus could conceivably upset the mechanisms controlling lymphocyte reactivity so that they respond abnormally to antigens to which they should remain tolerant. This idea receives some support from experiments in which animals stimulated with certain microorganisms (e.g. tubercle bacilli or corynebacteria) or the products of organisms (e.g. bacterial endotoxin) do not develop the expected immune tolerance when these antigens are administered in a way which would induce tolerance in normal animals.

The human autoimmune disease systemic lupus erythematosus is characterized by anti-DNA antibodies and immune complexes containing DNA present in the kidneys (Fig. 9.1). Tubular structures resembling the nucleocapsids of myxo or para-myxoviruses have been found by electron microscopy in the endothelial cells of renal glomeruli and occasionally in the

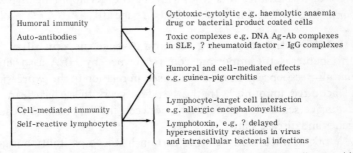

Fig. 9.1 Scheme showing pathogenic mechanisms in autoimmune disease with examples of disease states in each category.

lymphocytes and joint tissues. Similar particles have been found in the tissues of patients with a number of other diseases in which autoantibodies are found (thyroiditis, myasthenia gravis, sclero-derma and dermatomyositis). A relationship between these findings and the pathogenesis of these diseases has not yet been established and is complicated by the difficulty in distinguishing between immune reactions directed against virus specified antigens and host antigens (autoantigens).

Stimulation of pre-existing B cells. Another explanation for the development of auto-antibodies has recently been put forward (Table 9.1) – stimulation of a pre-existing population of lym-phocytes (B cells) capable of making anti-self antibodies. In the mouse, cells making anti red cell auto-antibodies can be induced to proliferate by the administration of substances with adjuvant activity (p. 45) e.g. certain corynebacteria and *B. pertussis*. Evidence indicating the presence of such lymphocytes was provided some years ago by a number of immunologists including the author, who described a variety of naturally occurring auto-antibodies in the serum of rodents. The availability of techniques such as immunocyto-adherence and localized haemolysis in gel (p. 41) have now allowed the identification of the lymphocytes producing the auto-antibodies and thus put the earlier observations on a much firmer footing. It is a matter of speculation at present whether any human auto-immune state is a result of stimulation of these anti-self reactive lymphocytes. Recent evidence suggests that B cells lose tolerance more readily than T cells and that T cells tolerant to self may be bypassed by presenting auto-antigens to B cells in a sufficiently immunogenic form perhaps combined with adjuvants as discussed above. If as seems possible, the antibodies produced were of low affinity this would favour the development of toxic complexes with results as described on page 101.

HLA, immune response genes and disease susceptibility

In Chapter 4 the important role performed by HLA associated immune response genes was discussed in relation to the expression of acquired immunity. In the last few years there has been an extensive search for associations between the expression of these genes and disease states.

Work in mice indicates that certain histocompatibility antigen linked immune response genes, appear to predispose to murine autoimmune thyroiditis and susceptibility of mice to lymphocytic-choriomeningitis virus infection. Theses studies suggest that products of histocompatibility linked immune response genes, possibly expressed as receptors on T lymphocytes, may be important factors in genetic susceptibility or resistance to autoimmunity, infection and neoplasia.

In man there have been very extensive studies of disease states and histocompatibility antigen types and the results appear to indicate that certain diseases, such as systemic lupus erythematosus, psoriasis and Graves disease, show a low but possibly significant association between the presence of disease and particular histocompatibility antigen types when compared to the normal population. For example, SLE patients carry the W15 HLA antigen in about 36 per cent of cases, whereas the normal population show this antigen in 10 per cent of individuals. The W27 antigen and the A8 antigen likewise appear in 50 per cent or less of patients with psoriasis and Graves disease, respectively, compared to 8 and 22 per cent in control population. The HLA antigen showing a relationship to Graves disease appears to vary in different populations, whilst associated with the A8 antigen in Caucasians, in Japan the association is with the BW5 antigen. In contrast to this low association, ankylosing spondylitis, acute chronic hepatitis and gluten enteropathy show a high association between the disease and particular HLA antigens. Eighty-eight per cent of ankylosing spondylitis patients have the W27 antigen, 68 per cent active chronic hepatitis patients have the A8 antigen and 88 per cent of patients with gluten enteropathy have the A8 antigen. In contrast the normal population express the W27 antigen in 8 per cent of persons and A8 in just over 20 per cent. The fact that none of these associations are absolute indicate that there are other factors, even possibly other genes, not linked to the HLA system. In support of this possibility the disease multiple sclerosis shows a much closer association with the MLC (mixed lymphocyte culture reaction) gene complex (70 per cent compared to 15 per cent of controls) than with the HLA antigen (A7), where only 36 per cent of patients carry this antigen compared to 25 per cent of controls; thus the MLC gene is closer to the susceptibility factor than HLA 7. Environmental factors such as exposure to viruses may also be required for a susceptible individual to develop the disease and the disease itself may have more than one aetiology.

There is little doubt that as further knowledge is gained of the HLA system, especially of the associated immune response genes (p. 84) and their role in the immune response itself, more insight will be gained into resistance or susceptibility to a variety of neoplastic, autoimmune and infectious diseases of man.

The pathogenesis of autoimmune disease
There is even more uncertainty in this area than exists with respect to the underlying abnormalities and stimuli which induce the autoimmune response.

Autoimmune diseases can be classified as **hypersensitivity** reactions on the basis of the definitions given in Chapter 6. These immune reactions, in contrast to those involved in protection from infectious disease, actually bring about severe and sometimes fatal reactions affecting the individual's own tissues and cells. The hypersensitivity reactions are divided into four types and three of these encompass autoimmune reactions.

Cytolytic or cytotoxic (type 2) reactions
The foremost of the autoimmune conditions in this category is autoimmune haemolytic anaemia. Here the antibodies are of two main types: (1) antibodies of the IgM class which agglutinate the patient's own red cells in the cold; (2) antibodies of the IgG class

which do not usually bring about direct agglutination of the red cells but can be detected by the Coombs test (p. 182) using an antiglobulin serum.

The anaemia is caused largely by the removal of antibody-coated cells in the spleen or the liver. Only rarely does lysis or agglutination take place to any extent in the circulation and involve the uptake of serum complement. Whilst normal red cells survive with a half life in the circulation of just over three weeks, in this form of anaemia they are unlikely to have a half life of more than one week.

Other forms of haemolytic anaemia exist including drug-induced types and those involving infective agents such as mycoplasma. Drugs involved include penicillin, phenacetin, quinine and α methyldopa. The anaemia is brought about by the reaction of antibody with the drug linked as a hapten to the red cell surface resulting in haemolysis. The precise details of the haptenic groups responsible for antigenic stimulation and their linkage to the red cell surface are uncertain. In mycoplasma infections the IgM cold agglutinins react with a widely distributed red cell antigen known as the I antigen.

Drug-induced agranulocytosis and thrombocytopoenia have also been described in which the leucocytes or platelets are destroyed by antibody directed at a complex of the drug and cell surface structures. Sedormid purpura has already been mentioned (p. 100).

Toxic-complex (type 3) reactions
Complexes of antibody and tissues antigens, particularly nuclear antigens (Fig. 9.1) are the cause of glomerulonephritis in a number of autoimmune states, notably in a disease known as systemic lupus erythematosus where a wide range of anti-tissue antibodies is found, and in the similar type of disease of NZB mice. Complexes of antinuclear antibody and nuclear antigen, together with complement, can readily be demonstrated in the glomerular capillaries. The glomerular basement membranes become thickened and secondary changes develop in the renal tubules with progressive renal failure. The role of toxic complexes has been extensively studied in mice infected with lymphodytic chorio-meningitis virus (see p. 127). Some strains of mice develop toxic complex nephritis whilst others do not. Current evidence suggests that toxic-complex reactions are most likely to occur in strains of mice that produce low affinity antibodies and thus fail to eliminate antigen effectively. Clearance of immune complexes has been shown in rabbits and monkeys to be related to the number of antigen and antibody molecules in the complex. In strains of mice prone to develop toxic-

complex nephritis low affinity antibodies are produced and thus the complexes would have poor lattice structure (p. 175) and not be cleared from the circulation by phagocytic cells as effectively as larger aggregates.

Cell-mediated (type 4) reactions

There is no doubt that in both man and experimental animals the development of a number of autoimmune states is paralleled by the finding of cell-mediated reactions of the delayed hypersensitivity type as demonstrated by skin tests using tissue antigens. Whether the diseases are actually caused by immune reactions mediated by lymphoid cells is a matter of conjecture. Support for the role of cells in the disease process comes from studies in an experimental autoimmune disease known as autoimmune allergic encephalomyelitis. This is brought about by immunization of animals with brain homogenate in Freund's complete adjuvant and paralysis follows demyelination of motor nerve fibres. The disease can be transferred in inbred strains of rats by the injection of lymphoid cells from affected animals to normal animals. The same type of transfer has been performed in autoimmune thyroiditis. In the latter condition it is proposed that the sensitized lymphocytes produce a surface injury to the cells of the thyroid acini and this allows the cytotoxic antibody frequently present in the serum of affected subjects, to enter the cell and react with intracellular antigens.

That there may be an interaction between cell-mediated immunity and a humoral antibody is emphasized by work on autoimmune orchitis in guinea-pigs. Animals injected with a purified testis homogenate in Freund's complete adjuvant develop cell-mediated immunity (as shown by the development of delayed hypersensitivity on skin testing) but no circulating antibody or testicular lesion. When these animals are injected with anti-testis antibody (from a guinea-pig injected with testis homogenate in incomplete Freund's adjuvant, i.e. without tubercle bacilli) orchitis can be shown to develop. This interpretation is supported by the finding that anti-testis antibody enters the seminferous tubules (as shown by the indirect fluorescent antibody method, p. 186) at the same time as cell-mediated immunity first appears (Fig. 9.1). Antibody-dependent cell-mediated cytotoxicity is described on page 105. The possibility that this form of reaction occurs in autoimmune states is supported by *in vitro* experimental work, but its role *in vivo* remains to be established.

Other diseases associated with autoimmune states

There is a large reservoir of diseases in which some form of autoantibody has been found but where neither the stimulus for autoantibody formation nor the role, if any, of immune reactions has been elucidated.

Among these conditions is rheumatoid arthritis in which an IgM antibody called rheumatoid factor is present in the serum. This antibody is detected *in vitro* by its ability to agglutinate red cells or latex particles which have been coated with IgG globulin (p. 195). The rheumatoid factor does not appear to be directly involved in the pathogenesis of the disease and no satisfactory explanation has been offered to account for its pathogenesis. The possibility has been suggested that infective agents are involved, such as mycoplasma or chronic infective bacterial agents, and there are reports of the isolation of such agents from rheumatoid joint arthritis in man and in a number of other species. One suggestion is that the infective agent may modify the lymphoid tissues so that there is a failure of the normal tolerance control mechanisms (p. 64). Experimental arthritis can be induced in rats by the injection of Freund's complete adjuvant containing killed tubercle bacilli. This is a polyarthritis with mononuclear cell infiltration similar to the arthritis found in a human illness known as Reiter's syndrome, the main features of which are urethritis and arthritis and which may occur in the presence of a mycoplasma infection.

Recent evidence suggests that there may be an IgG form of rheumatoid factor present in both the blood and joint fluid of rheumatoid patients as well as the IgM type and that injection of autologous purified IgG into previously unaffected joints can induce acute arthritis. Further evidence suggesting that an antigen-antibody reaction is taking place is provided by the low complement levels found in patients' joint fluid and the presence of immune complexes.

Rheumatoid factors react with the Fc fragment of IgG (rabbit or human) but not with the Fab fragment. Rheumatoid factors are sometimes found in patients with diseases other than rheumatoid arthritis. These include systemic lupus erythematosus, Sjögrens syndrome, scleroderma, lymphoproliferative disease and in certain persistent bacterial, protozoal and viral infections. Even healthy subjects sometimes have low titres of the factor in their serum particularly in the older age groups.

The mechanism underlying the appearance of these rheumatoid (anti-globulin) factors is not clear. In chronic infections it is conceivable that the factor is a response to antigenic determinants on the IgG molecule that are exposed when IgG antibody complexes with the infective agent. In the healthy individual a low titre of rheumatoid factor may perhaps serve a physiological function as a way of clearing degraded immunoglobulin molecules arising during infective or inflammatory processes.

Antibodies as a consequence of tissue damage

In considering the role of autoantibodies as a possible cause of autoimmune disease it should be remembered that antibodies of IgM type, directed at subcellular antigens, can be readily induced by various forms of tissue damage. These arise secondarily to the damage and appear to have no role in perpetuating it. Antibodies of this type have been shown in the author's laboratory and can readily be induced in rats by the injection of the hepatotoxic agent carbon tetrachloride, and it was subsequently found that normal rats, mice and hamsters have some IgM anti-tissue antibody in their serum. A possible physiological role for these antibodies is suggested by the finding *in vitro* of a chemotactic effect on rat polymorphs of a mixture of the antitissue antibody and its antigen. Thus the antibody might be responsible for initiating a phagocytic cell clearing process to deal with the breakdown products of normal cell turnover.

Recent evidence indicates that IgG antibody existing in the normal individual seem to be able to recognize glycoprotein determinants which appear on aged red blood cells. These determinants are exposed following the loss of sialic acid groups from the outside of the cells on ageing. Their exposure can be reproduced experimentally by treatment with neuraminidase. The IgG antibodies bind to the exposed glycoprotein and enable the attachment of the red cell to the Fc receptors (p. 14) on a macrophage. The aged red cell is then phagocytosed and destroyed by the lysosomal enzymes of the macrophage.

All autoantibodies are therefore not necessarily autoregressive, although the history of immunity and protection inculcates the idea of antibodies acting solely as aggressive agents.

FURTHER READING

Asherson, G. L. (1968) The role of micro-organisms in auto-immune responses. *Progr. Allergy.*, **12**, 192.

Asherson, G. L. (1968) Auto-antibody production as a breakdown of immune tolerance. In *Regulation of the Antibody Response*, p. 68, ed. Cinader, B. Springfield, Illinois: Thomas.

Burnet, F. M. (1959) *The Clonal Selection Theory of Acquired Immunity*. Cambridge University Press.

Dumonde, D. C., Steward, M. W., Glass, D. N., Maini, R. N. (1973) Immunology and the rheumatic diseases. *Brit. J. hosp. Med.*, **9**, 51.

Glynn, L. E. & Holborrow, E. J. (1964) *Auto-immunity*. Oxford: Blackwell.

Humphrey, J. H. & White, R. G. (1969) *Immunology for Students of Medicine*, p. 600. Oxford: Blackwell.

Irvine, W. J. (1967) Immunobiology of the thymus and its relation to auto-immune disease. In *Modern Trends in Immunology*, 2, p. 250, ed. Cruickshank, R. & Weir, D. M. London: Butterworth.

Levy, J. A. (1974) Autoimmunity and neoplasia: the possible role of C-type viruses. *Am. J. Clin. Path.*, **62**, 258.

Marmion, B. P. (1976) A microbiologist's view of investigative rheumatology. In *Infection and Immunology in the Rheumatic Diseases*, ed. Dumonde, D. C., p. 245. Oxford: Blackwell.

Marmion, B. P. & MacKay, J. M. K. (1977) Rheumatoid arthritis and the viral hypothesis. Bayer symposium VI. *Experimental Models of Chronic Inflammatory Diseases*, p. 188. Berlin: Springer-Verlag.

McDevitt, H. C., Bodmer, F. (1974) HL-A, immune response genes and disease. *Lancet*, **1**, 1269.

Moller, G. (1975) HLA and disease. *Transplant Rev.* **22**, 2.

Samter, M. (1965) *Immunologic Diseases*. Boston: Little Brown.

Talal, N. & Fyek, Moutsopoulos (1976) Autoimmunity. In *Basic and Clinical Immunology*, eds. Fudenberg, H. H., Stites, D. P., Caldwell, J. L. & Wells, J. V. Los Altos: Lange.

Trentin, J. J. (1967) *Cross-reacting Antigens and Neo-antigens (with Implications for Auto-immunity and Cancer Immunity)*. Baltimore: Williams & Wilkins.

Turk, J. L. (1969) *Immunology in Clinical Medicine*. London: Heinemann.

Weir, D. M. & Elson, C. J. (1969) Anti-tissue antibodies and immunological tolerance to self. *Arthr. and Rheum.*, **12**, 254.

World Health Organization (1977) Immune complexes in disease. Report of a WHO scientific group. *Wld Hlth Org.*, Technical report series no. 606.

10

Immunohaematology

Knowledge of blood groups in man and animals has been very closely associated with the development of the science of immunology. Differences between the red blood cells of animals were first noted in goats as early as 1900 when Ehrlich and Morgenroth immunized 'a strong male goat' with nearly a litre of blood obtained from three other goats. The serum which they obtained from the immunized goat lysed the cells of all but one of the nine goats they tested. However, to Ehrlich the most important finding was that the cells of the immunized goat itself were completely unaffected. This proved to him that an animal would not produce autoantibodies against its own tissues and so destroy itself. It was left to Karl Landsteiner, who made the same observations in humans, to take up the detailed study of these antigenic differences. Landsteiner's important work on the immunological determinants of antigenic specificity stems from this period and still stands today as of fundamental value to our understanding of antigens. Studies in blood group serology have led to the development of a large variety of techniques which have wide application to immunological problems outside this field. Notable amongst these is the antiglobulin test devised by Coombs and his associates, by means of which enormous advances have been made in many branches of immunology. Study of the development of blood group antibodies in serum has thrown light on the mechanisms underlying the formation of natural antibodies. Apart from these contributions to the understanding of immunological problems, information on blood groups has important implications in genetics and in forensic studies.

Blood groups

ABO antigens and isoantibodies
The ABO blood group system was described as a result of Landsteiner's demonstration of four distinct groups of aggluti-

nation reaction between human red blood cells and normal human serum. The differences in agglutination were due to the presence or absence of two antigens A and B on the red cell membrane. The four combinations which result from this are: (1) the presence of A antigen in the absence of B – group A cells; (2) the presence of B antigen in the absence of A – group B cells; (3) the presence of both A and B antigens – group AB cells; and (4) the absence of both A and B antigens – group O cells.

The sera of individuals also contain natural antibodies able to react with, and agglutinate if present in sufficient concentration, the cells of other individuals of different blood group.

These natural antibodies or **isoantibodies** are formed shortly after birth and appear to be stimulated by immunization with A and B antigens derived from the normal bacterial flora of the gut. Antigens with blood group specificity are widely distributed in nature (see also p. 22).

From a consideration of the phenomenon of immunological tolerance and the fact that an individual is tolerant to 'self' antigens (chap. 9) it can be seen that an individual will respond only to an antigen to which he is not already tolerant. Thus an individual with blood group A cells will be tolerant to the A antigen and will therefore respond only to the B antigen derived from the gut flora. The same holds for blood group B individuals who can respond only to the A antigen.

Thus individuals of blood group A will have isoantibodies of blood group B specificity, i.e. anti-B antibodies, and blood group B individuals will in the same way have anti-A isoantibodies. Blood group O individuals whose immune system will not have developed tolerance to either A or B antigens will have, as would be expected, both anti-A and anti-B isoagglutinins.

The blood group antigens A and B occur not only in the red cells but are widely distributed in the tissues with the exception of the central nervous system. Just under 80 per cent of individuals also have one of these antigens (corresponding to their blood group) in the tissue fluids and secretions (except CSF). Chemical studies on these antigens recovered in quantity from ovarian cyst fluid show them to be glycoproteins and that the difference between A and B substances is determined by the nature of a single saccharide attached to the terminal sugar of the glycoprotein chain. Group O individuals secrete a glycoprotein (H-substance) which is probably the basic chain structure material from which A and B substances are derived by the addition of the specific saccharides (p. 24).

Blood transfusion in relation to ABO groups

Transfusion of an individual with red cells from an individual of a different group results in exposure of the transfused cells to an isoagglutinin – anti-A or anti-B – and except in the case of O cells which carry neither the A nor the B antigen, the cells will be destroyed with resulting haemoglobinaemia and haemoglobinuria. Although it is clearly best to administer blood only of the same group as the recipient, in an emergency group O cells can be given. Although the plasma of a group O individual (sometimes called a **'universal donor'**) contains anti-A and anti-B isoagglutinins, these are so diluted by the recipient's plasma (a pint of blood would be diluted about 1 in 12) to have only a negligible effect except when large quantities of blood have to be administered. Group O individuals whose serum contains anti-A and anti-B isoagglutinins cannot accept blood of any group except O. Since an individual of group AB has neither anti-A nor anti-B isoantibodies he can accept blood of any of the four groups and has therefore been called a **'universal recipient'**.

This relatively straightforward scheme is unfortunately slightly complicated by the existence of a number of subgroups of A (probably five in all). However, only A_1 and A_2 are of importance as far as transfusion is concerned. The frequency of occurrence in Caucasians of the six different ABO groups is shown below.

Blood Group	Frequency	Isoantibodies
O	43.5%	Anti-A ($+$Anti-A_1), Anti-B
A_1	34.8%	Anti-B
A_2	9.6%	Anti-B (occasionally Anti-A_1)
B	8.5%	Anti-A ($+$Anti-A_1)
A_1B	2.5%	None
A_2B	0.8%	None (occasionally Anti-A_1)

The Rhesus blood group system

This system is the next most important system to the ABO groups. The Rh blood group antigens are present in the red cells of 85 per cent of Caucasians and 94 per cent of Negroes. The most common of the Rhesus antigens are C, c, D, d, E, e, and the table shows some of the various combinations which can exist and their frequency in Caucasians.

Genotype		Frequency	
CDe / cde	–	31.7%	⎫
CDe / CDe	–	16.6%	⎬ Rh-positive
CDe / cDe	–	11.5%	
cDE / cde	–	10.9%	⎭
cde / cde	–	15.1%	Rh-negative

The Rhesus group of an individual must be taken into account for transfusion purposes. Of these antigens D is the most potent although immunization by D and at the same time by the C or E antigens can occur. A variant of D named D^u has been described and cells carrying this antigen are not agglutinated by routine anti-D sera. For transfusion purposes recipients carrying the D^u antigen are considered to be Rh-negative, whilst donors in this category are regarded as Rh-positive.

Rhesus incompatibility

The clinical importance of the Rhesus groups lies in the ability of the red cells of a Rhesus-positive fetus to immunize its Rhesus-negative mother. Immunization usually takes place following the trauma of parturition with the result that the maternal immune response does not develop until a **second** pregnancy. The maternal anti-Rh antibody is passed to the new fetus via the placenta and causes haemolytic destruction of its erythrocytes. This condition is known as **haemolytic disease of the newborn** or erythroblastosis foetalis. Since the original description of the disease it has been found that blood group antigen systems other than the Rh system can be responsible for the condition. For example a group O mother can occasionally be immunized by fetal antigens if the father is A_1, A_1 B or B.

The serious nature of haemolytic disease of the newborn necessitating complete exchange of the infant's blood (exchange transfusion) to remove the maternal antibody, has now been alleviated by a rather ingenious immunological manoeuvre. This is based on the observation that attempted immunization by an antigen in the presence of its specific antibody tends to inhibit synthesis of the antibody to the injected antigen. It is known, for example, that immunization of infants is best delayed for a few months after birth to allow the levels of maternal antibody to fall.

In the case of a recognized Rhesus incompatibility it is now the practice to give a small dose of potent anti-Rh antibody to immunized Rh-negative mothers within three days after delivery of an Rh-positive infant. The antibody appears to inhibit the response to the Rhesus antigen, possible by diverting the cells carrying the antigen from the antibody-forming tissues or perhaps by a direct 'feedback inhibition' effect on the antibody-forming cells. This treatment has been very successful in clinical trials and the future outlook is very hopeful so that the disease may soon become of only historical interest (Fig. 10.1).

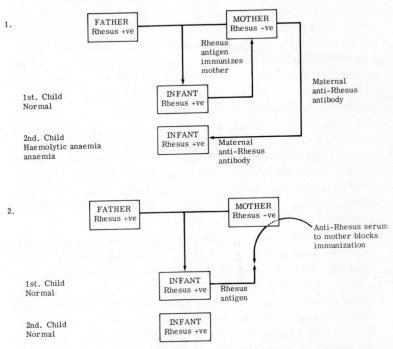

Fig. 10.1 Scheme showing consequence of immunization of Rhesus – ve mother by Rhesus antigen of Rhesus + ve child. Prevention obtained by injection of anti-Rhesus serum after delivery of first child.

The detection of anti-Rh antibodies

After the recognition of the association between haemolytic disease of the newborn and Rhesus immunization it soon became apparent that the standard method of demonstrating anti-Rh antibody – by direct agglutination of a saline suspension of Rh-positive cells by serum from an immunized mother – was not able to show up the presence of antibody in one-half to two-thirds of sera tested. A solution to the problem was found by the substitution of a dilute protein solution, e.g. bovine albumen, for the normal saline diluent. Visible agglutination could then be readily demonstrated in the majority of cases. The form of serum antibody responsible for agglutination demonstrable only in protein diluent, became known as 'incomplete' antibody in contrast to the saline-active 'complete' antibody. The incomplete antibody was thought of initially as univalent, having only one antibody-binding site, but it has now been shown to be IgG antibody of normal bivalent structure (p. 47); the complete anti-red cell antibody, on the other hand, has been shown to be IgM in nature. It seems that the smaller molecular weight IgG antibody is not readily able to link together red cells in suspension unless the mutually repellent effect of red cells, which normally keeps them in suspension in a saline medium, is reduced by altering their surface charge by the addition of protein. In contrast the much larger, multivalent IgM antibodies have a considerably greater chance of bringing about agglutination.

Another very important method for demonstrating incomplete antibodies is the Coombs antiglobulin test. An antiserum is prepared in rabbits against human immunoglobulins and this is used to react with Rh-positive cells, coated with human incomplete antibody, bringing about their agglutination simply by linking together the molecules of human globulin still attached to the red cells (p. 182 and Fig. 12.9).

One of the advantages of this method is that it can be used to detect the coating *in vivo* of Rh-positive cells by small amounts of antibody. After the cells have been thoroughly washed they are mixed with the anti-human globulin serum which will bring about agglutination of cells with human globulin attached to their surface. This form of the test is known as the 'direct Coombs test'. Another form of the test is used to detect incomplete anti-Rh antibodies in the serum of a patient who has been immunized against Rh antigens. Rh-positive cells are simply mixed with the patient's serum and if anti-Rh antibody is present the cells will be agglutinated by the subsequent addition of an anti-human globulin serum. This variation is known as the 'indirect Coombs test'.

Maternal responses to other fetal antigens

In addition to responding to the Rhesus antigen the mother can respond to other blood group antigens, and mothers lacking the A or B red cell antigen who carry a fetus possessing such antigen will probably develop raised levels of anti-A or anti-B isoagglutinins. Such sera are useful for blood typing purposes as are sera containing anti-HLA antibodies which are often found in multiparous women and which can be used for leucocyte typing. Spermatozoa, although they carry histocompatibility antigens, rarely seem to immunize. Immunization of the mother to fetal antigen probably occurs following passage of fetal blood (by small haemorrhages) into the maternal bloodstream and occurs more frequently as pregnancy progresses. Maternal lymphocytes can be found that have become sensitized to fetal and trophoblast antigens as detected by *in vitro* tests for cell-mediated immunity. Chorionic gonadotrophin hormone is believed to play an important role in protecting the fetus and is produced in quantity by the trophoblast, and there may be other maternal serum factors involved in protection of the fetus; in late pregnancy the numbers of circulating T lymphocytes are reduced, although the cause of this is not understood.

Other blood group systems

In 1927 Landsteiner described two human antigens, M and N. The use of antisera against these antigens can divide individuals into three types, half having the MN genotype and 28 per cent and 22 per cent respectively having MM and NN genotypes. A further antigen was later found, the S antigen, and the group is known as the MNS blood group system. This group is of limited clinical importance although a few instances of haemolytic disease of the newborn have been reported due to incompatibility of these antigens.

Landsteiner's P antigen is noteworthy because a naturally occurring anti-P cold agglutinin is found in a large proportion of the 20 per cent of individuals who are P-negative. Amongst a number of blood group systems described including those of Lutheran, Kell, Lewis, Kidd, Duffy and Diego, special mention should be made of the Lewis system because naturally occurring antibodies to Lewis antigens are frequently found in human serum. They sometimes act as cold agglutinins and have been found occasionally to be the cause of haemolytic transfusion reactions. These antigens are unique in that they are not part of the red cell structure but are soluble antigens found in body fluids, which adsorb on to the red cell surface.

Antigens of blood leucocytes and platelets

As has been discussed in the section on transplantation antigens, blood leucocytes in man carry the major histocompatibility antigen system HLA. The appearance of antibodies against donor leucocytes and also platelet antigens is a common finding after blood transfusion. This results in rapid destruction of the transfused cells and although immunization occurs more frequently than anti-red cell immunization the consequences are less dangerous.

Leucocyte and platelet groups fall into two types: those which they share in common with red cells, and those which are restricted to leucocytes and platelets and other tissue cells. The blood group antigens A and B are the main antigens shared with erythrocytes. The important antigenic group limited to leucocytes, platelets and other tissue cells is the HLA system.

A reaction between anti-leucocyte isoantibodies and transfused leucocytes often gives rise to febrile transfusion reactions and their incidence can be correlated with the number of transfusions given. Although these reactions are not usually severe they can be a disadvantage to patients for whom repeated transfusions are necessary. In this situation the simplest solution is to remove the majority of leucocytes from the blood by separation of red cells which can be readily sedimented by the addition of gelatin. This is preferable to the complex serological procedures required to assure compatibility of leucocytes.

The transfusion of fresh platelets is of value in patients suffering from haemorrhagic disorders due to thrombocytopoenia, and although theoretically, selection of compatible platelets is desirable, in practice platelets are usually obtained from a small number of donors, if possible related to the recipient.

The HLA system of antigens is of considerable current interest to immunologists because of their importance as histocompatibility antigens. Unfortunately the HLA system appears to be a most complex system but with wide implications in immunology. It is the equivalent of the H-2 system in the mouse and of the other main histocompatibility systems known to exist in other mammalian species (see p. 84).

Between 15 and 20 more or less well-defined antigens have been identified in the HLA system, and more than 100 phenotypes have been found within this system. Despite these complexities as more experience is gained in the grouping procedures (leucoagglutination by a panel of antisera), and supplies of suitable antisera become more widely available, it seems likely that by accumulating a list of available fully typed donors, and with improvements in storage and preservation of tissues it may eventually become possible to select from amongst the many possible variations a suitable donor for each recipient.

FURTHER READING

Bulletin of The World Health Organization (1967) The suppression of Rh-immunization by passively administered human immunoglobulin (IgG) anti-D (anti-Rh_0). *Bull. Wld Hlth Org.*, **36,** 467.

Dausset, J. & Colombani, J. (1967) White cells and platelets in transfusion immunology. In *Modern Trends in Immunology*, 2, p. 314, ed. Cruickshank, R. & Weir, D. M. London: Butterworth.

Dodd, B. E. & Lincoln, P. J. (1975) *Blood Group Topics.* Vol. 3 in *Current Topics in Immunology*, ed. Turk, J. L. London: Arnold.

Race, R. R. & Sanger, R. (1968) *Blood Groups in Man.* 5th edition. Oxford: Blackwell.

Stern, C. M. (1975) Feto-maternal relationships. In *The Immune System*, eds. Hobart, M. J. & McConnell, I. Oxford: Blackwell.

11

Malignant disease

In discussing the general biological significance of immune reactions in maintaining the integrity of the cellular systems of the body, Burnet points out that in man, in whom more than 10^{14} cells are constantly reproducing, there is sufficient evidence to make it likely that at any given genetic locus an error occurs with a frequency in the range of 10^{-5} to 10^{-7} per replication. This means that in the cell population there must be many millions of errors or mutations occurring every day of life. It seems inconceivable that complex and long-lived multicellular animals could have evolved unless some means of dealing with this eventuality had been developed. Recently, however, doubt has been expressed on this view and it has been suggested that 'this daily development of malignant cells is not supported by the experimental evidence, and that spontaneous malignant transformation *in vitro* appears to be dependent more on cell-to-cell interactions than to be an intrinsic property of single cells.'

The role of immunological mechanisms in the suppression of malignant cells has been appreciated since the work of Paul Ehrlich at the beginning of the century, but it is only in the last ten years or so that immunologists have begun to unravel the details of the immunological processes underlying the control of tumours, the antigenic changes in tumour cells themselves, and the extent and activities of the immune response arising as a result of these changes.

Evidence for the role of immune mechanisms
Mention is made in Chapter 8 of the increased incidence in thymectomized mice of tumours induced by chemical carcinogens and viruses. This seems likely to be due to a deficiency of the cell-mediated immune mechanisms which lie under the control of the thymus (p. 77). These neonatally **thymectomized** animals are unable to reject incompatible tissue grafts and do not give delayed hypersensitivity reactions of the tuberculin type. These activities

depend on intact cell-mediated, thymus-dependent immune reactivity and it is the absence of this reactivity which allows tumour cells to grow unhindered.

The experimental evidence in support of this view is conflicting. Thymectomy of mice does appear to increase the incidence of skin tumours to certain chemical carcinogens (polycyclichydrocarbons) and of tumours induced by DNA viruses. However, early thymectomy seems to have no significant effect on development of spontaneous tumours in mice and there are reports of a decreased incidence of tumours, such as mouse mammary carcinoma following thymectomy. It thus appears that the effects of thymectomy are variable and depend to some extent on other factors, such as the agent responsible for tumour development.

Another example where deficiency of the cell-mediated immune mechanisms is associated with tumour formation is in a condition known as **graft-versus-host** disease. This condition is produced in mice by injecting spleen cells into an unrelated recipient, the reaction of the spleen cells against the host resulting in destruction of its lymphoid tissues. This can be demonstrated by using two inbred strains of mice, e.g. CBA and C57 Black, and injecting the spleen cells of one of the parents into the offspring of such a mating. CBA cells injected into a CBA/C57B recipient will recognize the C57B component of the host-lymphoid cells as foreign but will not be themselves rejected because the recipient itself carries the CBA antigens.

The destruction of the recipient's lymphoid tissues and thus its cell-mediated immune response, produces a defect in the control of neoplastic cell proliferation and the mice frequently develop tumours of the lymphoid tissues having many of the features of Hodgkin's disease of the human.

A herpes virus (Epstein Barr) has been isolated from the human lymphoid tumour known as **Burkitt's lymphoma** and it has been proposed that the tumour is of virus origin induced perhaps in the way described above. Recent evidence in patients with Burkitt's lymphoma has added considerable support to the significance of cell-mediated immune mechanisms in the control of the tumour. Only one of 12 patients on skin testing with extracts of their own tumour cells have positive delayed hypersensitivity reactions. However when the tumour growth was suppressed with cyclophosphamide, skin tests became positive in seven of the twelve indicating a recovery of the cell-mediated immune mechanisms which is associated with remission of the tumour.

Serological studies have demonstrated a strong association

between the presence of high titres of antibody to EB virus in both Burkitt's lymphoma and postnasal carcinoma. However, antibody to the virus is widespread throughout the world and association can be found with a number of diverse disease states. The virus can be found not only in leucocytes of patients with Burkitt's lymphoma but also in leucocytes of patients with infectious mononucleosis and even in some normal individuals. The virus appears to be able *in vitro* to **transform** leucocytes into virus-containing cells capable of continuous growth. The virus appears to have a predilection for cells of the lymphoid organs and it cannot yet be excluded that the virus is a 'passenger' trapped within lymphoid cells present in the tumour rather than the prime cause of the tumour. Recent evidence suggests the possibility that the herpes viruses may act indirectly on cells by activating a latent RNA tumour virus. Ultraviolet light irradiated herpes simplex virus, whilst unable to destroy mouse cells, resulted in the activation of an endogenous virus similar to the RNA tumour viruses.

There is as yet no firm evidence that tumours in humans are caused by viruses; recent work in America suggesting the possible role of a virus as a cause of mammary carcinoma has proved to be ill-founded. The possible involvement of a transmissible viral agent in human sarcomas has been proposed in the last few years. A common surface antigen has been found on sarcoma cells derived from bone, cartilage, fat and muscle and induces a detectable antibody response in patients' serum. This antigen can be transferred to normal human fibroblasts by exposing them to the filtered culture medium from sarcoma cells. That the antigen is transmittable to other individuals is suggested by the finding that cohabitants of sarcoma patients have the anti-sarcoma antibody in their serum.

Carcinomas of the gastrointestinal tract can be shown to contain an antigen absent from normal adult gut cells but present in those of embryos. The antigen termed **carcinoembryonic antigen** (CEA) has been found in the blood of patients with such tumours and their lymphocytes appear to be able *in vitro* to act against their cultured tumour cells in contrast to control lymphocytes that have no effect.

A somewhat disturbing result of the use of anti-lymphocytic serum (ALS) in man for immunosuppression in tissue transplantation (p. 114) is the small but significantly increased incidence of tumours in such individuals; it seems probable that this is due to suppression of immunological surveillance mechanisms. It is also interesting to note that various chemical immunosuppressive drugs and X-rays, acting like ALS on the lymphoid tissues, are in many instances carcinogens as well as immunosuppressive agents. In recent experiments performed to test the effects of immunosuppression by ALS on tumour incidence, once again the results have not been clear cut. As in the situation with thymectomized mice, local tumour incidence following chemical carcinogens was increased after ALS treatment. In studies of the development of spontaneous leukaemias in ALS treated mice, there are reports of both increased and decreased tumour incidence and the problem so far remains unresolved.

The incidence of cancer in man is highest at the two extremes of life and it is just at these times that the immune system is least efficient. All these observations point to the probable important role played by the intact immune mechanisms in maintaining the body free of undesirable mutant neoplastic cells.

There is considerable discussion amongst immunologists concerning the particular cells of the immune system that may be responsible for '**surveillance**' mechanisms to deal with neoplastic cells or host cells altered in other ways. The emphasis has shifted from a central role for the thymus dependent (T) lymphocyte (partly because of the conflicting experimental evidence discussed above) to a role for the **macrophage** which can readily be shown *in vitro* to have cytotoxic effects against tumour cells (see p. 170). Tumours are often heavily infiltrated with macrophages, and transfer of such cells in an activated state (see p. 170) to mice with experimental tumours has been shown to lead to tumour suppression. Macrophages undoubtedly have the ability to recognize and bind to their surface (with and without antibody) various foreign materials such as bacteria and altered cells (e.g., red cells), and it is not unreasonable to suppose that this ability might extend to recognition of neoplastic cells.

Tumour antigens

It can be deduced from the foregoing discussion that for the immunological system to react against tumour cells, these cells must be changed in some way so that they are no longer recognized as self. That this is indeed so is substantiated by many examples of tumours which have been found to develop **new antigens** as part of their cell structure. There are two types of antigenic change: (1) where the specificity of the new antigen is dependent on the inducing agent such as a virus, and (2) tumours induced by chemical carcinogens in which the antigenic change induced by the same carcinogen in two different animals is different in each case. The carcinogen methylcholanthrene has been reported to induce different antigenic changes in cells even in the same animal if the chemical is applied to two separate areas.

There are numerous examples of tumour formation which seem to be associated with these changes. The SV_{40} virus induces tumours in monkeys, the Rous sarcoma virus in chickens and the polyoma virus in mice. The tumours induced in mice by the polyoma virus have recently been shown to consist of two sorts of cells – cells that are malignant on introduction into another mouse and cells that do not survive transplantation. It seems possible that the latter cells are destroyed by the immune system because they carry recognizable foreign antigens on their surface. When cells of the non-transplantable variety are cultured *in vitro* variants appear which have lost their antigenicity and can thus transfer the tumour. This raises the possibility that attempts to eliminate malignant cells by increasing the immune reaction against them may result in the 'selection' of 'non-antigenic' variants which would allow the tumour to spread.

The tumour-specific antigens are comparable to the weak histocompatibility antigens (p. 108) and their strength has been found to vary for different aetiological groups. Methylcholanthrene-induced sarcomas in mice have been found to be more strongly antigenic than similar sarcomas induced by dibenzanthracene. Among the virus tumours, Moloney virus-induced lymphomas of the mouse are quite strongly antigenic whereas the Gross agent induces a similar tumour with very weak tumour specific antigens. Consistent with the finding that the specificity of tumour antigens varies even with one chemical carcinogen is the finding that the strength of these antigens varies also.

Having established that antigenic changes occur in neoplastic cells and that immunological processes are apparently involved in the body's reaction to tumours, the question is how in fact does any tumour grow and spread throughout the body in the face of the body's immune reaction? Some of the factors which tip the balance in favour of tumour growth have already been discussed in relation to central defects of the immune response.

Another important factor is that the tumour-specific antigens are often not strongly antigenic and the degree of immunity developed is insufficient to cause the rejection of a rapidly growing tumour. In experiments in mice, with primary tumours induced by chemical carcinogens, it has been shown that if a mouse is pre-immunized with tumour cells (inactivated by X-irradiation) the animal can then develop a state of immunity to transfer of living tumour cells provided that the number of transferred cells is not too large to overcome the induced immunity.

The abnormal social behaviour of tumour cells is well known in that they generally fail to form stable intercellular adhesions. It would not be surprising if the interaction between tumour cells and cells of the lymphoid system would likewise be abnormal leading to escape of the tumour cell from the potentially cytotoxic effects of lymphocytes.

Another way in which tumours could escape the attention of lymphocytes sensitized to the tumour antigens is by the **shedding** from the tumour of excess antigen. Such antigen present in the serum of patients with malignant disease is believed to account for the inhibitory effect of such serum on lymphocyte cytotoxicity for the tumour. Free tumour antigen or antigen-antibody complexes could conceivably 'blindfold' sensitized lymphocytes thus preventing them from identifying and attaching to tumour cells themselves.

Implications in cancer therapy

The classical treatment for carcinoma of the breast and many other tumours is the radical surgical removal of the neoplastic tissue and much of the surrounding tissue, including the lymph glands of the area.

It is now recognized that this treatment sometimes enhances the spread of secondary deposits, and it is thought that this might be due to removal of lymphoid tissues involved in the immune response to the antigens of the tumour, and possibly also to diminution in the antigenic stimulus to the immune system. The balance is thus tipped in favour of remaining tumour cells which can proliferate unchecked. In addition it should be remembered that mammary carcinogenesis almost certainly also involves the interplay of a variety of non-immunological factors – hormonal, genetic and possibly viral.

A number of ways have been proposed of inhibiting tumour growth by enhancing the immune response to the tumour antigens either by active immunization with tumour antigens or by non-specifically stimulating the lymphoid tissues. This area is fraught with ethical and practical difficulties but a few partially successful, albeit heroic, experiments have been tried in man.

In one small series in America, malignant tissue was interchanged between pairs of patients with 'incurable' tumours. After allowing sufficient time for an immune response, leucocytes from the immunized individual were injected into the original donor of the tumour tissue. Clinical benefit was claimed in 5 of the 14 patients

involved, one patient having complete remission with the disappearance of the numerous secondary tumour deposits of a
malignant melanoma with no sign of a recurrence after one year.

Agents known to stimulate the cells of the lymphoid tissues in a
non-specific manner have come into vogue in the last few years as a
form of cancer immunotherapy. This interest derives from the work
in France of Mathé who has employed BCG (p. 137) treatment as
part of the therapy of acute lymphoblastic leukaemia in children.
The length of the remissions in such cases appeared to be
prolonged. The possible value of **non-specific stimulation** of the
immune system is pointed to by some recent work with such an agent,
Corynebacterium parvum. Mice injected with *C. parvum* and given
vigorous antitumour chemotherapy showed complete remission in
up to 70 per cent of mice with a chemically induced sarcoma. The
effect was found only when the two treatments were combined.
Other experiments in mice showed that BCG was most effective if
given a week or more before the injection of tumour cells. This
indicates that the treatment is not likely to be effective in the presence
of an established tumour unless some steps are taken to reduce the
tumour mass by drug or X-ray therapy.

Corynebacterium parvum and BCG injected directly into mouse
tumours can be shown dramatically to suppress tumour growth.
The effect appears to be largely due to a cell-mediated immune
response to the antigens of the microorganisms, in which lymphoid
cells are attracted to the injection site in large numbers and appear
to act not only on the bacterial antigens but also on the surrounding
tumour cells.

Another effect of these organisms is to '**activate**' the macrophages
of the injected animal in such a way that they can be shown *in vitro* to
become cytotoxic for cultured tumour cells. It is difficult to be sure
that this effect operates *in vivo* but it is possible, at least where tumour
cells are circulating in the blood stream or free in a body cavity, that
activated macrophages could capture and destroy them.

In conclusion it seems possible that immunotherapy may have
an important role in the future treatment of malignant disease. It
seems likely to be most effective when the tumour mass is small or
can be reduced by chemotherapy. The spontaneous disappearance
of tumours and complete recovery of patients with widespread
cancer does on rare occasions happen and is usually explained as
divine intervention. A more readily acceptable explanation of such
phenomena is that for some reason the balance between tumour
growth and the immune reaction against it has been tipped in favour
of the immune response.

FURTHER READING

Bengesh-Melnick, M. & Batel, J. S. (1974) In *The Molecular Biology of Cancer*, ed. Busch, H. New York: Academic Press.

Burnet, Sir Macfarlane (1962) *The Integrity of the Body*. London: Oxford University Press.

Burnet, Sir Macfarlane (1970) *Immunological Surveillance*. London: Pergamon Press.

Chirigos, M. A. (1977) *Control of Neoplasia by Modulation of the Immune System*. New York: Raven Press.

Currie, G. A. (1975) Immunology of malignant disease. In *Medical Oncology*, ed. Bagshawe, K. D. Oxford: Blackwell.

Gell, P. G. H., Coombs, R. R. A. & Lachmann, P. J. (Eds.) (1975) *Clinical Aspects of Immunology*. 3rd edition. Oxford: Blackwell.

Hamilton Fairley, G. (1971) Immunity to malignant disease in man. *Brit. J. hosp. Med.*, **6**, 633.

Fenner, F. (1968) *The Pathogenesis and Ecology of Viral Infection*. New York: Academic Press.

Stutman, O. (1975) Immunodepression and malignancy. *Adv. Cancer Res.*, **22**, 261.

Trentin, J. J. (1967) *Cross-reacting Antigens and Neo-antigens (with Implications for Auto-immunity and Cancer Immunity)*. Baltimore: Williams & Wilkins.

Turk, J. L. (1969) *Immunology in Clinical Medicine*. London: Heinemann.

12

The interaction of antibody with antigen

An antibody, as has been pointed out, is an immunoglobulin molecule secreted into the tissue fluids from lymphoid cells which have been exposed to a foreign substance – an antigen. An antigen may be potentially harmful, such as bacterium or virus, or it may be a harmless bland substance such as foreign serum protein. The antibody can combine only with antigen which is identical or nearly identical with the inducing antigen and not with unrelated antigens. When molecules of antibody and antigen are brought together in solution, they interact with each other by the formation of a link between an antigen-binding site on the immunoglobulin molecule – part of the Fab fragment – and the particular chemical groupings which make up what is termed the antigenic determinant of the antigen molecule. The molecules are held together by **non-covalent intermolecular forces** which are effective only when the antigen-binding site and the antigenic determinant group are able to make close contact. The better the fit the closer the contact and the stronger the antigen-antibody bond, these factors determining what is often called the **affinity** of the antibody molecule; antibodies of varying combining quality exist and the overall tendency to combine with antigen is the average ability of the antibodies to combine with antigen or the average intrinsic association constant. This can be calculated experimentally by application of the concepts of chemical equilibria to antigen-antibody interactions. Studies of this type have shown that the affinity of antibodies increases as immunization proceeds and that the dose of antigen can influence the quality of antibody (see p. 69).

The methods used for the detection of antigen-antibody reactions in the laboratory fall into two functional groups: first, procedures designed to elucidate .the cytodynamics of antibody formation which involve the study of the behaviour of single cells or small populations of cells; the second group, which is the subject of the present discussion, concerns the detection and quantitation of

secreted antibody circulating in the blood or present in the tissue fluids.

The methods used here range in their application from highly specialized studies of the physico-chemical aspects of antigen-antibody interaction to widely used procedures designed to aid in the diagnosis of disease.

Primary interaction and secondary effects

In practical terms, the union of antibody with antigen can be detected at two different levels. The first level is that following **primary union** of the two reactants and usually requires that one or other reactant is labelled with a suitable marker such as a fluorescent dye or a radioactive isotope. A simple example of this is the microscopic localization in a tissue of a particular microorganism utilizing an antiserum prepared against the microorganism and labelled with a dye that fluoresces under UV light. A widely used method in experimental immunology makes use of the fact that immunoglobulins are insoluble in 50 per cent saturated ammonium sulphate. The test developed by Farr uses antigen labelled with ^{131}Iodine that is mixed with antibody containing serum and left to equilibrate. Ammonium sulphate solution is then added to the mixture resulting in the precipitation of the antibody together with any labelled antigen bound to it. The unbound antigen remains in solution (only antigens that are themselves soluble in 50 per cent ammonium sulphate can be used in this form of the test). The quantity of isotope labelled antigen bound to the salt precipitated antibody is then estimated by placing the washed precipitate in radioactive counting equipment. This sensitive and useful technique is a measure of the capacity of an antiserum to bind antigen.

The second level at which antigen-antibody combination can be detected depends on the development, after primary union, of certain changes in the physical state of the complex, resulting in precipitation or agglutination of the components or, alternatively, in the activation of non-antibody components such as serum complement or histamine from mast cells. Reactions of this type occurring subsequent to primary union are termed **secondary phenomena.** This discussion is concerned with the principles of a few of these secondary phenomena which are in common use.

Secondary effects; interpretation and applications. Before considering these reactions individually, it is important to be aware of the difficulties in interpreting results of such tests. The initiation and development of the secondary phenomena constitute a complicated series of events involving many variables such as the type of antibody taking part, the relative proportions of antibody and antigen, characteristics of the antigen molecule, presence of electrolytes, inhibitory substances and unstable components.

Despite these formidable difficulties, the widely and long used secondary phenomena such as precipitation, agglutination and complement fixation have an important role to play as aids in the diagnosis of disease and in the identification of microorganisms.

The secondary phenomena, as already indicated, can bring about several readily observable changes when carried out *in vitro* and these are used in tests to demonstrate the presence of antibody in the sera of patients suffering from infectious disease, or producing an antibody response to cell antigens as might, for example, occur after incompatible blood transfusion, tissue grafting or in autoimmune states.

Reactions of this type can also be used to identify antigens in the tissues or body fluids and, for example, would be utilized for blood grouping, tissue typing or the identification of microorganisms.

Among the most important of these reactions are **precipitation**, which occurs between antibody and antigen molecules in soluble form; **agglutination**, in which the antibodies directed against surface antigens of particulate materials such as microorganisms or erythrocytes, link them together in large clumps or aggregates; and **complement fixation** in which antibody molecules, after reaction with antigen, activate the complex blood components that make up serum complement.

In addition to these widely used serological tests, a number of other effects of antigen-antibody interaction are of medical importance. These include **neutralization** tests used for example in virus identification, **immobilization** tests with bacteria and protozoa and **skin tests** for the reaginic antibody characteristic of anaphylactic states.

Precipitation

Optimal proportions. As a result of the interaction of antibody and antigen molecules in solution, complexes of the two types of molecule will form and precipitation may occur depending on the relative concentration of the two reactants. If a series of tubes is set up (Fig. 12.1), each containing a constant amount of antiserum, and decreasing amounts of antigen are added to the tubes in the row, a haziness will start to appear in the tubes gradually increasing to clearly visible **aggregates** or **precipitates**. The amount of pre-

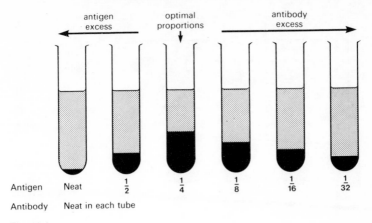

Antigen   Neat $\frac{1}{2}$ $\frac{1}{4}$ $\frac{1}{8}$ $\frac{1}{16}$ $\frac{1}{32}$

Antibody   Neat in each tube

Fig. 12.1

cipitation will be seen to increase along the row, reaching a maximum and then falling off with the lower antigen concentration. The tubes where most precipitate appears contain the **optimal proportions** of antigen and antibody for precipitation and the proportions are constant for all dilutions of the same reagents. The composition of the precipitate varies with the original proportions of the antibody and antigen; if antigen is in excess the precipitate will contain relatively more of this component and similarly more antibody if it is present in excess. As can be seen from Figure 12.2, on the antigen excess side of optimal proportions less precipitate appears and this is due to the inability of the antigen-antibody complexes formed to link up to other complexes and so make a large aggregate or lattice which will appear as a visible precipitate (tube 1, Fig. 12.2). Large aggregates of antibody and antigen can form best under conditions of optimal proportions where the antibody and antigen proportions are such that after initial combination of the molecules, free antigen-binding sites and antigen determinant groups remain, enabling the complexes to link up into a large lattice formation (as in tube 2 of Fig. 12.2). In antibody excess all the free determinants of the antigen molecule are soon taken up with antibody, so that very little linking can take place between the complexes (as in tube 3 of Fig. 12.2).

Applications. The precipitin test can be carried out in a quantitative manner by estimating the protein content of the precipitate at optimal proportions. The qualitative test is much more widely used and is of considerable value in detecting and identifying antigens,

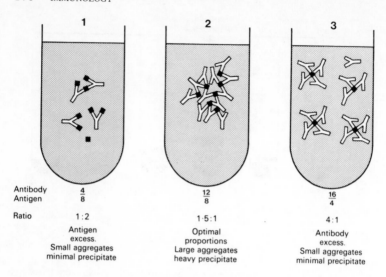

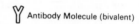 Antigen Molecule (can react with 4 antibody molecules)   Y Antibody Molecule (bivalent)

Fig. 12.2

having applications in the typing of streptococci or pneumococci. This is done by layering an extract of the organism over antiserum. After a short while, a ring of precipitate forms at the interface (this is called the ring test). The technique is also used in forensic studies and in detecting adulteration of foodstuffs. A modification of the test in which precipitation is allowed to occur in **agar gel** is very widely used for detecting the presence of antibody in serum or antigen in unknown preparations, and is valuable for showing the identity of different antigen preparations (Fig. 12.3). A concentration gradient forms in the gel, the concentration of a substance decreasing as the molecules diffuse away from the well in which they were placed. **Precipitin bands** form in the gel in the position where the antigen and antibody molecules reach optimal proportions after diffusion.

When a large number of different antigens are present in a solution, it is difficult to separate the precipitin bands for each of the antigen-antibody reactions by the simple gel-diffusion method just described. In such a situation, a variation of this method can be used to identify the individual components. This modification is particularly valuable in analysing a multicomponent system such as serum. The individual components of serum are first separated by

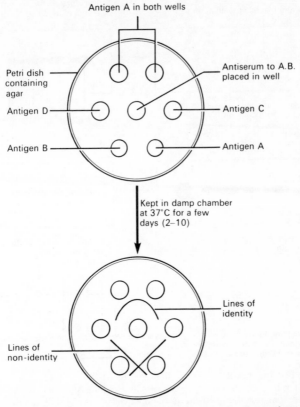

Fig. 12.3 Immunodiffusion or gel diffusion test. Wells are cut in a layer of agar in a Petri dish. Antiserum and antigen solutions are placed opposite each other in the wells and after allowing a few days for diffusion to take place precipitin bands will form where antibody and antigen meet in suitable proportions (optimal proportions). No reactions take place with antigens C and D as the antiserum in the central well contains antibodies only for antigens A and B. Lines of identity as formed between the two A wells enable the technique to be used for identifying unknown antigens.

electrophoresis in agar gel and an antiserum, prepared against the serum, is allowed to diffuse towards the separated components, resulting in the formation of precipitin bands (Fig. 12.4). This method, known as **immunoelectrophoresis**, is particularly valuable for showing the presence of abnormal globulin constituents in the serum of patients with myelomatosis and other serum protein abnormalities.

A microimmunodiffusion test with wells cut in a layer of agar on a microscope slide is a convenient modification of the Petri dish method. This procedure has come into wide use for the detection in

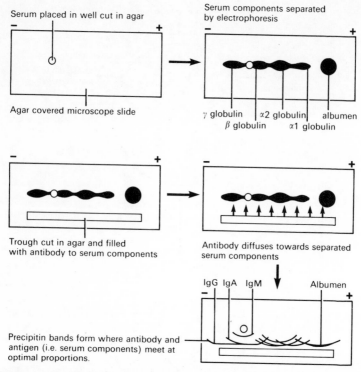

Fig. 12.4 Immunoelectrophoresis. The antigen, for example, serum, is placed in a small well cut in a layer of agar on a microscope slide. A direct current is applied and differential migration of the serum components takes place. (They are not normally visible in the agar and will show up only if suitably stained.) After electrophoresis for an hour or so, a trough is cut longitudinally in the agar and an antiserum against the electrophoresed antigen is placed in the trough. The two components diffuse towards each other and precipitin bands form. These can be shown up more clearly by staining with a protein stain. This is a very powerful analytic technique and can show up about 30 different components in human serum compared with 4 or 5 by electrophoresis.

human serum of the **Australia antigen** which is associated with serum hepatitis. The routine screening of blood products by this technique using specific antisera prepared in animals is likely to become an important laboratory test in the prevention of serum hepatitis outbreaks.

Instead of placing antibody and antigen in separate wells and allowing them to diffuse towards each other, the antibody can be incorporated in the agar and the antigen placed in wells. This technique is known as **single radial immunodiffusion** and depends upon diffusion of antigen from the well until a point is reached where the concentration is optimal for precipitation to occur. Close to the antigen well the concentration of antigen will be high and although the antigen will combine with antibody in the agar, the complexes will be unable to form the large lattice structure necessary for precipitation to take place (Fig. 12.2) and will thus remain as soluble complexes. The precipition band that forms at optimal proportions of antigen and antibody will show up as a ring around the antigen well. The distance the ring forms from the antigen well will be dependent on the concentration of the antigen in the well. In practice the **diameter** of the ring is measured around a well containing an unknown concentration of antigen and this is compared with the diameter of the rings formed with known concentrations of the antigen thus enabling the estimation of the concentration of antigen in the unknown preparation. This technique is widely used to estimate the quantity of the various immunoglobulin classes in human serum samples. An antiserum to a particular immunoglobulin class (e.g. IgG) is incorporated in the agar and the test serum sample is placed in a well. The diameter of the precipition band that forms after incubation is then compared to the diameter obtained with standard IgG preparations of known concentration. The diameters of the rings with the **standard** IgG preparations (e.g. 3 or 4 dilutions of a known concentration) can be plotted graphically against the concentration of IgG and the diameter obtained with the unknown sample can be read off against concentration on this reference graph (Fig. 12.5).

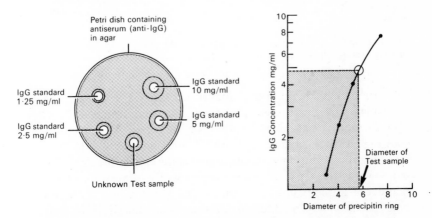

Fig. 12.5 Diagram of single radial immunodiffusion plate with antiserum incorporated in agar and antigen dilutions and test sample in wells. Reference Graph drawn using 3 concentrations of antigen standard showing the diameter of precipitin ring obtained with each concentration (●). Diameter of unknown sample (○) when plotted enables determination of its antigen concentration.

Agglutination

In this reaction the antigen is part of the surface of some particulate material such as a red cell, bacterium or perhaps an inorganic particle (e.g. polystyrene latex) which has been coated with antigen. Antibody added to a suspension of such particles combines with the surface antigens and links them together to form clearly-visible aggregates or **agglutinates** (Fig. 12.6). In its simplest form an agglutination test is set up in round-bottomed test tubes or perspex plates with round-bottomed wells and doubling dilutions of the

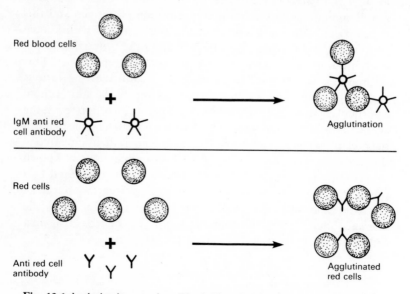

Fig. 12.6 Agglutination reaction. The IgM molecule with at least five antigen-binding sites is particularly effective in bringing about agglutination.

antiserum are made up in the tubes (neat, 1:2, 1:4, 1:8, etc). The particulate antigen is then added and after incubation at 37°C agglutination is seen in the bottom of the tubes. The last tube showing clearly visible agglutination is the end point of the test. The reciprocal dilution of the antiserum at the end point, e.g. 1/256 is known as the **titre** of the antiserum and is a measure of the number of antibody units per unit volume of serum, e.g. if the end point occurs at a 1/256 dilution of the antiserum and if the test has been carried out in 1 ml volumes, the titre of the serum is 256 units per ml of serum. One practical difficulty of importance in agglutination tests is the occasional inhibition of agglutination in the first tubes of an antiserum dilution series, agglutination occurring only in those tubes containing more dilute antiserum. This is known as the **prozone phenomenon** and is probably, in part, due to the stabilizing effects of high protein concentration on the particles, the protein coating the particles, increasing their net charge and so bringing about increased electrostatic repulsion between individual particles, thus opposing the efforts of the antibody molecules to link the particles together. However, once the protein concentration is reduced by dilution the antibody molecules can then exert their aggregating effect and bring about agglutination. The agglutination reaction has been shown to require the presence of electrolytes in the suspending medium and is usually performed for this reason at physiological salt concentration.

Applications. One of the classical applications of the agglutination test in diagnostic bacteriology is the **Widal test** used for the demonstration of antibodies to salmonellae in serum specimens taken from suspected enteric fever cases. Agglutination is the basic technique used in blood grouping, the A, B or O group of the red cells under test being determined by agglutination with a specific antiserum – an anti-A serum for example will agglutinate A cells but not B or O cells. Red cells and inert particles such as polystyrene latex can be coated with various antigens and suitably coated particles are used in a variety of diagnostic tests such as thyroid antibody tests using thyroglobulin-coated cells or latex particles. Hormone-coated red cells or inert particles are used in many hormone assay procedures which are based on the inhibition of the antibody-induced agglutination of the hormone-coated particles by hormone added in the sample under test (Fig. 12.7). Tests of this type are in wide use in pregnancy diagnosis.

Certain viruses, e.g. the myxoviruses causing influenza and mumps, have the property of bringing about agglutination of red cells (haemagglutination). **Inhibition of haemagglutination** by antibody in patients' serum is a widely-used diagnostic procedure. The presence of antibody in the patient's serum is thus detected by its ability to link with virus particles and prevent them from bringing about agglutination of the red cells (Fig. 12.8).

IgM antibodies capable of agglutinating human red cells (including those of the individual producing the antibody) between 0 and 4°C are sometimes found in certain human diseases including primary atypical pneumonia, malaria, trypanosomiasis and acquired haemolytic anaemia.

The presence of antibody globulin on a red cell may not result in

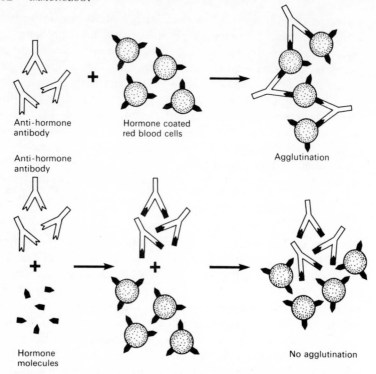

Fig. 12.7 Principle of hormone assay by agglutination inhibition. Red cells coated with hormone are agglutinable by anti-hormone antibody. The addition to the antiserum of a test sample containing free hormone will block the antigen-binding sites and prevent agglutination. The test can be carried out quantitatively by comparing the activity of a known standard hormone preparation with the test sample.

direct agglutination of the cells, for example in some Rh-negative mothers with Rh-positive infants or in acquired haemolytic anaemia. It is, however, possible to show that the red cells are coated with antibody by using an **antiglobulin** serum (produced in the rabbit by injecting human globulin) which will bring about agglutination of the cells (Fig. 12.9). This is the basis of the Coombs test which is a very widely used serological procedure.

Complement fixation
The fact that antibody, once it combines with antigen, is able to activate the complement system is used as a way of showing the presence of a particular antibody in a serum, e.g. the **Wassermann** antibody in syphilis, or in identifying an antigen such as a virus.

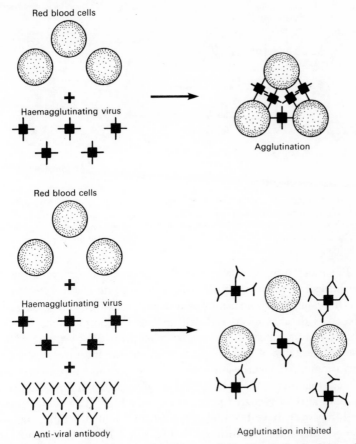

Fig. 12.8 Virus haemagglutination inhibition test. Red cell agglutination is brought about by a variety of viruses (see text). This can be inhibited by mixing the virus with anti-viral antibody as shown in the diagram. The test can be quantitated by comparison of serial dilutions of virus alone and virus-antibody mixture.

The complement system consists of a group of at least nine serum factors of globulin nature present in the serum of normal individuals. The complement of most species will react with antibody derived from other species and guinea-pig serum is a common laboratory source of complement – some of the components of complement are heat labile and are destroyed by heating at 56°C for 20 to 30 minutes. The individual components of the complement system are taken up by the antigen-antibody complex in a particular order and destruction of the heat-labile components which are taken up early prevents the remaining components from taking part (see p. 16).

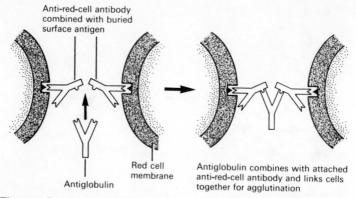

Anti-red-cell antibody combined with buried surface antigen

Antiglobulin

Red cell membrane

Antiglobulin combines with attached anti-red-cell antibody and links cells together for agglutination

Fig. 12.9 Coombs antiglobulin test. The red cell antibody, probably because it is directed against an antigen situated deep in the cell wall, cannot link two red cells together for agglutination. The addition of an antiglobulin serum brings about agglutination by linking two attached immunoglobulins to one another.

For most antigens the reaction of the complement system with the antigen-antibody complex causes in itself no visible effect, and it is necessary to use an indicator system consisting of sheep red cells coated with anti-sheep red cell antibody. Complement has the ability to lyse the antibody-coated cells, probably by virtue of the esterase activity of one of the components acting on the red cell membrane. In a test the antibody, complement and antigen are first mixed together and after a period of incubation the indicator system, antibody-coated sheep cells, are added. The complement will, however, have been taken up during the incubation stage by the original antibody-antigen complex and will not be available to lyse the red cells. Thus, a **positive** complement fixation test is indicated by **absence of lysis** of the red cells whilst a negative test, with unused complement, is shown by lysis of the red cells (Fig. 12.10).

Applications. The classical complement fixation test is the Wassermann reaction used in the diagnosis of syphilis in which the test system consists of Wassermann antigen mixed with dilutions of the patient's serum in the presence of guinea-pig complement. After the antigen and patient's serum have had time to react and take up the limited amount of complement available in the system, the indicator system is added to show whether or not there is free complement. Controls are included to ensure that none of the reagents are anti-complementary (able to take up complement non-specifically as might, for example, occur with contaminated serum)

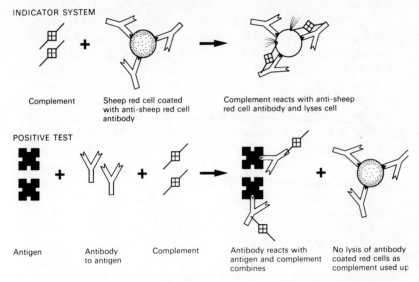

Fig. 12.10 Complement-fixation test. The indicator system (sheep red cells coated with antibody to sheep red cells) is normally lysed in the presence of complement (fresh guinea-pig serum) – top. If another antibody-antigen system is first mixed with the complement it will no longer be available to lyse the indicator system – bottom.

and positive and negative control sera are tested in parallel. Complement fixation tests are used routinely for detecting viruses in tissue cultures which have been inoculated with specimens of blood or tissue fluids from humans with probable virus infections.

Antigen-antibody reactions using fluorescent labels

The precise localization of tissue antigens or the antigens of infecting organisms in the body, of anti-tissue antibody and of antigen-antibody complexes was achieved by the introduction of the use of fluorochrome-labelled proteins by Coons and Kaplan in 1950. The adsorption of ultra-violet light between 290 and 495 mμ by fluorescein and its emission of longer wavelength green light (525 mμ) is used to visualize protein labelled with this dye. The technique is more sensitive than precipitation or complement fixation techniques, and fluorescent protein tracers can be detected at a concentration of the order of 1 μg protein per ml body fluid.

Applications. Some of the uses to which the technique has been put include the localization of the origin of a variety of serum protein components, for example immunoglobulin production by plasma cells and other lymphoid cells. The demonstration and localization in the tissues of antibody globulin in a variety of autoimmune conditions has been shown, including an anti-nuclear antibody in the serum of patients with systemic lupus erythematosus and thyroid auto-antibodies in the sera of patients with Hashimoto's thyroiditis. In the diagnostic field most human pathogens can be demonstrated by immunofluorescence and a tentative diagnosis may be made much sooner than by cultivation; the fluorescent method at present can be used to supplement rather than replace conventional methods.

There are two main procedures in use, the direct and indirect methods (Fig. 12.11). The **direct method** consists of bringing fluorescein-tagged antibodies into contact with antigens fixed on a slide (e.g. in the form of a tissue section or a smear of an organism), allowing them to react, washing off excess antibody and examining under the UV light microscope. The site of union of the labelled antibody with its antigen can be seen by the apple-green fluorescent areas on the slide. The **indirect method** can be used both for detecting specific antibodies in sera or other body fluids and also for

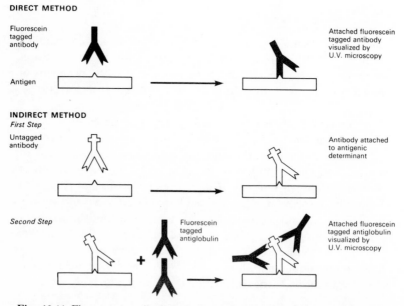

Fig. 12.11 Fluorescent antibody technique–direct and indirect methods. The indirect method can be seen to be more sensitive as two or more fluorescein-tagged antiglobulin molecules can be attached to each immunoglobulin molecule bound to its antigen.

identifying antigens. This method differs from the direct method in the use of a non-labelled antiserum which is layered on first, in the same way as described above. Whether or not this antiserum has reacted with the material on the slide is shown by means of a fluorescein-tagged **antiglobulin serum** specific for the globulin of the serum applied first. Such an antiglobulin serum can be used to detect antibody globulin in sera to a variety of different antigens which gives it a considerable advantage over the direct test; it is also more sensitive.

Other types of labelled antibody test have been developed on the same principles as the fluorescent methods. Horseradish peroxidase can readily be linked to antibody leaving the antibody still able to combine with its antigen. After this has occurred (e.g. in a tissue section layered with the peroxidase labelled antibody and then washed) the site of localization of the antibody can be visualized by conventional histochemical staining of the peroxidase using its substrate (the peroxidase reaction). Ferritin (an electron dense blood pigment) conjugated antibody has also been used in electron-microscope studies to show the localization of cell antigens.

Cytotoxic tests
Tests of this type are used in combination with red blood cell agglutination for studying histocompatibility antigen systems in tissue typing.

The cytotoxic test consists essentially of determining whether or not the **permeability** of cells changes after their incubation with antibody and complement (Fig. 12.12). Cytotoxic antibody after combination with the target cell will activate complement components and bring about changes in permeability of the cell membrane. The permeability changes can affect the ability of the cell to exclude a dye such as trypan blue which will penetrate the cell and be visible by simple microscopic examination.

Although the test is applicable to a wide range of nucleated cells and is the test of choice with blood leucocytes, it is rather less sensitive than the red cell haemagglutination tests and more laborious to perform.

Radioimmunoassay methods
Increasing use has been made over the last few years of immunologically based assay methods for the accurate quantitative estimation of **polypeptide hormones**. These methods offer a unique combination of specificity, precision and simplicity and are

NEGATIVE TEST—No antibody

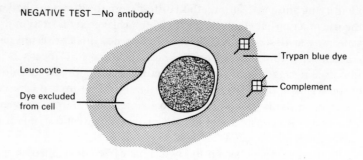

Leucocyte

Dye excluded from cell

Trypan blue dye

Complement

POSITIVE TEST—Antibody present

Complement reacts with antibody and makes cell membrane permeable to dye

Antibody

Trypan blue enters cell

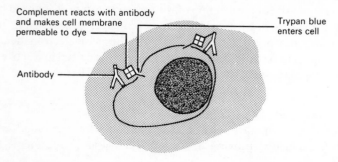

Fig. 12.12 Cytotoxic test.

already available for the assay of some 14 of the 20 or so polypeptide hormones in man.

The principle of the assay methods is that radio-iodine labelled (purified) hormone competes with the non-labelled hormone of a sample under test, for the anti-hormone antibody with which the labelled and non-labelled hormone are mixed. The more of the hormone in the test sample the less chance the labelled hormone has of combining with the limited number of antibody molecules that are available in the anti-hormone serum. Thus by measuring the quantity of labelled hormone combined with antibody (using isotype counting equipment) a measure of the hormone in the test sample can be obtained. The more labelled hormone combined with antibody the lower the hormone level in the test sample. The quantity of isotope labelled hormone complexing with the anti-hormone antibody varies inversely with the quantity of unlabelled hormone in the test sample.

In order to measure the amount of labelled hormone attached to antibody it is necessary to separate the hormone-antibody complexes from the mixture. A variety of methods have been developed to achieve this perhaps the most common being electrophoretic separation. Provided the **free** hormone has a different electrophoretic mobility from the antibody globulin then separation of hormone **bound** to antibody is straightforward. Other methods of separation depend upon the antibody being linked to an insoluble support (e.g. cellulose). The insoluble complex is then mixed with labelled and test hormone (tube 1, Fig. 12.13), allowed to interact

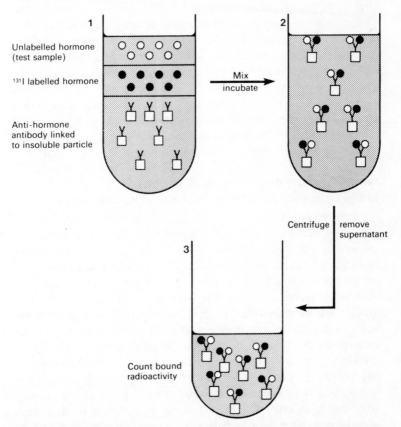

Fig. 12.13 Illustration of the use of antihormone antibody linked to an insoluble particle for the assay of the amount of hormone in a test sample. The quantity of ^{131}I labelled hormone complexing with the anti-hormone antibody varies inversely with the amount of unlabelled hormone in the test sample. A standard curve can be prepared using known concentrations of purified hormone in the same way as illustrated in Fig. 12.5, this will enable the result obtained with the test sample to be plotted and its concentration obtained.

(tube 2, Fig. 12.13) and later the unreacted hormone is removed and the amount of labelled hormone attached to the insoluble complex is measured (tube 3, Fig. 12.13).

An assay for IgE levels in serum has been developed using iodine labelled IgE and anti-IgE linked to cellulose, and assays using these principles are being developed for the detection of Australia antigen in human serum.

Immunoassays using enzyme-linked antibody or antigen

Labels other than radioactive isotopes and fluorescent dyes can be linked on to antibody or antigen molecules. There has been recent interest in the use of enzymes such as horseradish peroxidase or alkaline phosphatase linked to antibody or antigen molecules. The presence of the enzyme linked molecule is detected by means of the enzyme substrate and can be measured by spectrophotometry. Either the labelled antigen or the antibody can be attached to an insoluble support, such as plastic beads or plastic agglutination plates, and a number of convenient qualitative and quantitative assays are being developed for the detection of hormones, antigens of microorganisms or antibodies in a patient's serum. Assays of this type are known as enzyme linked immunosorbent assays (ELISA).

Some common diagnostic applications of antigen-antibody reactions in medical microbiology

Agglutination tests

The agglutination tests already referred to for the sero-diagnosis of salmonella infections is known as the Widal test. It is usual to test dilutions of the patient's serum against standard suspensions of somatic (O) antigen and flagellar (H) antigen of each organism likely to be encountered in the patient's environment. The test usually becomes positive with both suspensions, a week after the onset of the illness but may be weakly positive with one of the antigens even earlier. The titre in an acute infection rises to a maximum by the end of the third week. Complications in interpretation of the results may arise in patients who have been immunized with typhoid-paratyphoid vaccine (TAB). A **rising titre** may be of some help in diagnosing an infection; furthermore, some months after immunization the titre of O agglutinins tends to fall off leaving only H agglutinins. Normal sera sometimes have low titres of agglutinins for Salmonella organisms and this varies in populations in different parts of the world. These difficulties make the test of questionable diagnostic value and its use is now limited.

Another widely used agglutination test is the **Paul-Bunnell** reaction. This is used for the diagnosis of infectious mononucleosis in which agglutinins develop for sheep erythrocytes. Normal serum may agglutinate sheep cells in low dilutions and a titre of 128 is taken as suggestive and 256 as positive for the test. In some individuals who have received horse serum as a therapeutic agent (e.g. anti-tetanus serum) agglutinins develop for sheep cells because of the presence in the horse serum of an antigen very widespread in nature, known as the **Forssman** antigen. This antigen is present in the red cells of sheep and the cells of a number of other species, including the guinea-pig. The usual way of differentiating the two types of antibody is to mix the serum with minced guinea-pig tissue (usually kidney). This treatment will absorb out the anti-Forssman antibody leaving the anti-sheep cell antibody unaffected. Ox red cells which contain both the Forssman antigen and an antigen similar to that on sheep cells, which reacts with the Paul-Bunnell antibody, will absorb out both types of antibody.

Complement fixation tests
These tests, described on page 182 have wide application in the diagnosis of bacterial and viral infections. One of the most commonly used methods is the Wassermann test used in the diagnosis of **syphilis**. This reaction depends upon the fixation of complement by the patient's antibody after it has reacted with cardiolipin, an alcoholic extract (a phosphatide lipoid) from normal animal tissues, usually ox heart. Why antibodies against this material develop in syphilis is not clear. Some workers suggest that it results from autoimmunization with host lipids made antigenic in some way by the spirochaete (*Trep. pallidum*) responsible for syphilis whilst others believe that the spirochaete contains a cell wall antigen related to the tissue antigen (p. 22). Interpretation of the results of the Wassermann test is difficult and a final assessment depends on the results of both this and other serological tests and the clinical findings. False positive reactions are sometimes found in leprosy, malaria, sleeping sickness, tuberculosis infectious mono-nucleosis and other febrile diseases. Persistent **false positive** reactions are sometimes found in autoimmune haemolytic anaemia, systemic lupus erythematosus and liver cirrhosis. A commonly performed test is a slide flocculation test using cardiolipin mixed with the patient's serum. This test is preferred by many laboratories because of its simplicity as an alternative to the Wassermann test. It is known as the VDRL (Venereal Diseases Research Laboratory) slide test. When there is doubt a more specific test may have to be employed e.g. the treponemal immobilization test, in which motile

treponemata can be seen to be immobilized when examined microscopically after exposure to patient's serum. This test is, however, technically complicated and has largely been replaced by an indirect fluorescent antibody (p. 185) test (fluorescent treponemal antibody absorbed, FTA-ABS test). The test is highly specific and sensitive; it is able to detect antibody at all stages of syphilitic infection. The enzyme-linked immunosorbent assay (ELISA) described on page 190 has the potential for large scale application in syphilis serology.

Complement fixation tests are used widely in the diagnosis of virus diseases. The source of the antigen is usually the infected tissues of animals, or eggs, or infected tissue cultures. The virus is usually extracted from the tissues or cells by differential centrifugation or sometimes by purifying the virus by adsorbing it on to red cells and then eluting it later.

Haemagglutination-inhibition tests

Another useful procedure for the diagnosis of some types of virus disease is the **haemagglutination-inhibition** test. This depends on the fact that certain viruses, e.g. those of influenza, mumps and parainfluenza will agglutinate chicken, human and guinea-pig red cells (Fig. 12.8). Other viruses, e.g. the adenoviruses, agglutinate rat or monkey red cells; the reoviruses and many enteroviruses agglutinate human red cells. The test is performed by mixing the virus with the appropriate red cells in the presence of patient's serum. If antibodies to the virus are present the virus will be unable to bring about haemagglutination. These tests are very valuable because of their extreme specificity and their ability to distinguish antibodies to various substrains and variants of viruses, e.g. the influenza virus. The complement fixation test on the other hand is less valuable for detecting these fine differences.

LABORATORY INVESTIGATIONS IN CLINICAL IMMUNOLOGY

Increasing attention is now being paid in the clinical laboratory to the investigation of the role of immune reactions in the **pathogenesis** of disease and to methods of assessing the **functional status** of the immune system in situations where apparent immune dysfunction exists.

Many of the disease states in which immune reactions are believed to be involved in disease pathogenesis have been considered briefly in preceding chapters on hypersensitivity reactions and autoimmune states. Immune deficiency states are referred to in Chapter 5. This text is not to be intended to replace the many excellent textbooks dealing with the laboratory aspects of clinical immunology but to provide a simple outline of the main principles of this complex and difficult subject.

Investigation of hypersensitivity states

Antibodies in anaphylactic states

Hay fever and asthma sufferers characteristically have IgE antibodies in their blood. In 1921 Prausnitz and Küstner described a method for the detection of such 'reaginic' antibody performed by injecting a small quantity of serum from the hay fever patient into the skin of a normal subject. The IgE antibody fixes to the cells of the recipient close to the site of injection and when the antigen (or allergen) to which the patient is sensitive (e.g. a pollen extract) is injected at the site, an inflammatory response takes place due to the release of histamine from mast cells (see p. 95). The same type of reaction can be elicited in the patient by introducing a small quantity of dilute antigen into the skin (Prick test).

IgE antibodies can be quantitated by the radial immunodiffusion technique described on page 179. IgE directed at particular antigens can be assayed by coupling antigen to an insoluble material and mixing the complex with the patient's serum containing IgE antibody against the antigen. After allowing the binding of the IgE antibodies with antigen to take place, unbound serum proteins are washed away and the bound IgE antibody is detected with radio-labelled (^{125}I) anti-IgE antiserum.

Another procedure that can be used to detect sensitization to a particular antigen is to collect peripheral blood leucocytes from the patient and mix them with antigen. The lymphocytes will bind the antigen by their cell membrane receptors, as described on page 41, and the cells will be stimulated to transform in the way described on page 73. Macrophage migration inhibition tests have also been applied to detect sensitization to antigens. This procedure is described on page 74.

Another laboratory procedure as yet little used in clinical practice is the determination of the histocompatibility antigen type (p. 162) of the peripheral blood leucocytes. In studies in the United States an association has been found between the occurrence of allergy to ragweed antigen (antigen E) and HLA haplotypes. These studies have been confined so far to a small number of families. The association has been found to occur within particular families, making it possible to identify within a particular family the members at risk and likely to develop the particular ragweed allergy. If these studies are confirmed leucocyte typing may become a useful laboratory aid to the clinician.

Antibodies to inhaled organic material

A condition called 'extrinsic alveolitis' has been recognized in persons who inhale organic material such as fungal spores, dust from various birds or dust from mouldy hay or barley. The lung changes appear to be associated with IgG antibodies formed against the inhaled material and these antibodies are detected by gel diffusion precipitin tests, as described on page 177.

Pulmonary aspergillosis due to inhalation of spores of *Aspergillus fumigatus* sometimes develops in patients with asthma or with an old healed tuberculous cavity, and precipitating antibodies can be detected in their serum. *Candida albicans* respiratory infections can also result in similar antibodies.

Inhalation of *Micropolysporon faeni* from mouldy hay can result in a form of alveolitis known as farmer's lung disease, and mouldy barley containing *Aspergillus clavatus* can result in maltworker's lung disease. Gel diffusion tests for precipitating antibodies against antigenic extracts of the microorganisms have proved useful in the diagnosis of the conditions (see also p. 134).

Inhalation of antigens from birds is responsible for bird fancier's lung disease, and here again precipitating IgG antibodies can be detected against avian antigens. The antigens are present in bird serum, feathers and droppings and for the most reliable results material should be used from the particular species of bird to which the patient has been exposed – chickens, pigeons, budgerigars, parrots, and so on.

Antibodies against self-constituents (autoantibodies)

Organ (or tissue) specific autoantibodies

Autoantibodies against organ-specific antigens or non-organ-specific antigens are found in a wide range of disease states, as described in Chapter 9. Whilst their role, if any, in the disease process itself is not clear, their presence can be a useful guide as an aid in clinical diagnosis.

Amongst the more common organ-specific autoantibodies are those found in autoimmune haemolytic anaemia. Two main types of antibody have been found. (1) So-called 'warm antibodies' that combine at body temperature with red cells. These are usually of IgG class in contrast to IgM anti-red cell autoantibodies responsible for 'cold antibody' haemolytic anaemia that can be shown to agglutinate red cells at 4°C. The detection of these antibodies usually depends on the use of the Coombs antiglobulin test described on page 182. (2) Leucocyte and platelet autoantibodies have also been described in some rare disease states and are occasionally induced by drugs that combine with these blood components (p. 100).

Organ-specific autoantibodies have been described in the serum of patients with thyroiditis, adrenal disease, pernicious anaemia and disease of the salivary glands (Sjögren's syndrome). The main test here is the fluorescent antibody method (p. 185) with tissue sections of the appropriate tissue, but passive haemagglutination (p. 181) or gel diffusion tests are sometimes used in which red cells are coated with the tissue antigen or the antigen is placed in the wells for the immunodiffusion test (p. 177) with the patient's serum in opposite wells.

Non-organ-specific antibodies

In certain disease states such as rheumatoid arthritis and systemic lupus erythematosus (discussed in chap. 8) autoantibodies are found in widely distributed antigens not restricted to any one organ or tissue. Autoantibodies in this category are also found in various forms of chronic liver disease.

An agglutination test is widely used for the diagnosis of rheumatoid arthritis; the sera of 70 to 80 per cent of patients with this disease contain an IgM antibody which is able to combine with the IgG globulin from various species. Detection of the antibody depends on the agglutination of sheep red cells or inert particles (polystyrene latex) coated with IgG globulin. Sheep red cells, for example, may be coated with specific rabbit antibody and will then be agglutinated by the IgM antibody in the rheumatoid patient's serum. The antibody is known as **rheumatoid factor**. Occasional low titres (less than 16) are found in normal sera (2 to 5 per cent) and the test is not entirely specific for rheumatoid arthritis.

The fluorescent antibody test is the most commonly used method for the detection of the **antinuclear factor** (ANF) found in the majority of cases of systemic lupus erythematosus. Sections of tissue, e.g., rat liver, are used as the substrate and are layered with patient's serum. Binding of ANF to the liver cell nuclei is detected with fluorescein labelled antihuman immunoglobulin (see p. 186).

In a liver disease known as primary biliary cirrhosis most patients have antibodies against mitochondrial antigens. These are detected by the fluorescent antibody test with unfixed tissue sections or sometimes by complement fixation tests with rat liver mitochondria. In chronic active hepatitis, and transiently in just over half of patients with infective hepatitis, antibodies are found against smooth muscle actomyosin. The fluorescent antibody test is the method of choice using unfixed sections of rat stomach.

Immune deficiency states

The clinical and immunological aspects of these states are discussed in Chapter 5 and can be seen to involve one or more of the different components of the immune system: (1) the cells responsible for making circulating immunoglobulins, (2) the cells concerned with the cell mediated immune response and (3) the bone marrow stem cells. A wide range of laboratory tests are available to investigate the various forms of deficiency.

Immunoglobulin production. Assay of circulating immunoglobulins can be assessed qualitatively by electrophoresis and quantitatively by immunodiffusion tests. These latter tests are capable of identifying deficiencies of particular classes of immunoglobulin, as described on page 178.

The ability of the patient to make specific immunoglobulin can be tested by **active immunization** with, for example, a bacterial antigen such as tetanus toxoid and the antibody response measured by a tube precipitation test (p. 175).

The presence of the cells involved in the humoral immune response can be assayed by making use of the fact that the particular cells concerned – the B lymphocytes – have receptors on their surface for the Fc component of the Ig molecule and for the C3 complement component. In the test, sheep red blood cells coated with anti-sheep red cell antibody and complement (in non-lytic quantities) are mixed with peripheral blood leucocytes. The sheep red cells become attached to B lymphocytes by means of the Fc and C3 receptors (that combine with the antibody and complement on the red cell) forming 'rosettes' (p. 41). The proportion of leucocytes forming such rosettes gives an estimate of the number of B lymphocytes and is normally about 25 per cent of the lymphocytes in human peripheral blood.

Tests of the function of the cell-mediated immune system
Skin tests. The classical method for testing the responsiveness of the cells involved in cell-mediated immunity is the **delayed hypersensitivity skin test** described on page 103. The tuberculin response is the best known example. It is induced by the intradermal

injection of 0.1 ml of a 1:1000 dilution (or a greater dilution in a highly sensitive individual) of a protein extract of tubercle bacilli (purified protein derivative, PPD). The reaction is described on page 103; it is only one of a number of similar tests of delayed hypersensitivity such as that using lepromin (in leprosy) and brucellin (in brucellosis). One of the main uses of tests of this type is to detect sensitization to the relevant microorganism, as for example prior to the use of the BCG vaccine (p. 137) in the prevention of tuberculosis. Clearly in the presence of a positive tuberculin test immunization with the vaccine will not be called for. A negative reaction in an adult, particularly in one known to have previously shown a positive test, raises the possibility of a defect of the cell-mediated immune system, which in the adult would be likely to be secondary to some disease state affecting the lymphoid tissues such as Hodgkin's disease, multiple myeloma, leukaemia and lymphosarcoma.

Lymphocyte function tests. The thymus-dependent (T) lymphocyte has been pointed to as the main effector cell in cell-mediated immune reactions (chap. 4). The presence of the T lymphocyte in the peripheral blood can be detected very much in the same way as B lymphocytes can be detected. Instead of using antibody and complement coated sheep red blood cells as is required for B cells, sheep cells alone are all that is required. T lymphocytes have receptors for sheep erythrocytes and can thus form rosettes when the two types of cell are mixed together. Between 40 and 60 per cent of the human peripheral blood lymphocytes can form rosettes of this type.

Lymphocyte transformation. A particularly useful and widely used assay of lymphocyte function is the lymphocyte transformation test. This is usually carried out using plant phytohaemagglutinin (PHA) as the stimulating agent; the process is described in some detail on p. 73. In other situations a transformation test may be performed with specific antigens to which the individual is believed to be sensitized (e.g. tuberculin). In contrast to the use of PHA, which stimulates a high proportion of T lymphocytes, specific antigen will only stimulate those lymphocytes that are specifically 'committed' to the antigen in question and this is usually only a small proportion of the total T lymphocytes. A low level of lymphocyte transformation (when compared with control subjects), either with PHA or specific antigen, indicates impaired cell-mediated immunity (or perhaps absence of previous exposure to the antigen used), whilst increased transformation in the presence of a specific antigen may occur in certain hypersensitivity states, e.g. drug allergies (p. 104).

Migration inhibition. A modification of the macrophage migration inhibition test (see p. 74) using human peripheral blood leucocytes (instead of guinea-pig peritoneal macrophages) can be used in the assessment of cell-mediated immunity. Peripheral blood leucocytes are collected in a small capillary tube in the same way as described in the macrophage inhibition test and, when put in a culture chamber, grow out of the end of the tube in a fan shape. If, however, antigen, to which the cell donor has previously be sensitized, is put into the chamber the leucocytes fail to grow out of the tube. This inhibitory effect is believed to be due to a 'lymphokine' produced by the sensitized lymphocytes on exposure to antigen. This form of assessment of lymphocyte function has very much the same value as the transformation tests referred to above.

Tests of phagocytic cell activity. Defective phagocytic mechanisms are discussed in Chapter 5 and can be assayed in a variety of ways in the laboratory:

1. The ability of phagocytes to respond to a chemotactic agent (e.g. antigen-antibody complexes in fresh serum) can be measured by inducing the phagocytes to migrate from a chamber through a millipore membrane towards an outer chamber containing the Ag–Ab complexes and serum. The number of phagocytes that respond can be estimated by removing the membrane, staining it with a suitable stain and, under the microscope, counting the number of cells either in the process of passing through the membrane or on the outer side of the membrane.

2. The ability of phagocytes to ingest and kill microorganisms (e.g. staphylococci) or ingest inert particles such as latex or oil droplets can be determined by microscopic examination of cell preparations mixed with the microorganism or inert particle. Killing of microorganisms within phagocytes can be estimated by disrupting the cells (e.g. by distilled water) and counting the colonies of microorganisms that can be grown on a suitable nutrient agar plate.

3. The normal functioning of phagocyte lysosomal enzyme activity can be assessed by a dye reduction test using tetrazolium nitroblue. A defect on the part of the patient's cells can be detected by a failure of the leucocytes to reoxidize the reduced colourless dye to its blue colour. A deficiency of this function is characteristic of chronic granulomatous disease (p. 92).

The complement system. Changes in the levels of this complex group of serum protein constituents (see chap. 2) are often a reflection of an underlying disease process. **Raised** levels of the components are frequently found in acute inflammatory and infective disease states in conjunction with raised levels of 'acute phase proteins' such as C reactive protein.

Reduction in complement levels is a more useful guide to the understanding of disease pathogenesis and fall into two categories: (1) primary deficiencies – genetically determined deficiencies of complement components, and (2) secondary deficiencies – as a consequence of complement consuming antibody-antigen interactions or associated with renal or liver disease.

The genetically determined deficiencies are rare conditions, the best known of which is the deficiency of C1 esterase inhibitor (see p. 20). Very rare deficiencies of other components (C3, C1, C5) have been described.

The secondary deficiencies are much more frequently found and most often occur in renal disease such as post-streptococcal nephritis, in the nephritis of systemic lupus erythematosis and in chronic membrano-proliferative glomerulonephritis. Low levels also occur in serum sickness (immune complex disease), bacterial septicaemia, malaria and in various forms of liver disease.

In the laboratory two main types of assay are available: (1) functional tests of the haemolytic activity of the complement system, and (2) immunochemical estimation of the levels of individual complement components.

Haemolytic activity of the complement system is usually assayed by the method described by Mayer, which measures the number of 'units' of complement per ml of serum. A unit of complement is defined as the quality required to lyse 50 per cent of a standard sheep cell suspension, optimally sensitized with anti-sheep cell antibody. The volume, buffer components and incubation conditions are likewise defined. The test is sometimes referred to as a CH50 assay.

Estimation of individual components, whilst possible by assays of their functional activity, is usually performed by immunochemical methods utilizing specific antisera against individual components. The method of choice is the quantitative radial immunodiffusion test (p. 179) in which the antisera are incorporated in the agar and the serum specimens are placed in the wells. Commercially prepared plates are available for a wide range of complement components.

Other tests

A number of miscellaneous clinical immunological investigations are sometimes called for and include detection of circulating antigen-antibody complexes by precipitation with anti-C1q antiserum, examination of biopsy material for deposits of antibody or complement by immunofluorescence, estimation of cryoglobulins, radioimmunoassay for the presence of Australia antigen and characterization of monoclonal antibodies by immunoelectrophoresis or examination of bone marrow by immunofluorescence. Most of these procedures require specialized laboratory facilities not generally available in the routine clinical pathology laboratory.

FURTHER READING

Campbell, D. H., Garvey Justine, S., Cremer, Natilie E. & Sussdorf, D. (1963) *Methods in Immunology*. New York: Benjamin.
Cruickshank, R., Duguid, J. P., Marmion, B. P. & Swain, R. H. A. (1975) *Medical Microbiology*. 12th edition. Edinburgh: Churchill Livingstone.
Humphrey, J. H. & White, R. G. (1969) *Immunology for Students of Medicine*, p. 348. Oxford: Blackwell.
Nairn, R. C. (1969) *Fluorescent Protein Tracing*. 3rd edition. Edinburgh: Churchill Livingstone.
Nowotny, A. (1969) *Basic Exercises in Immunochemistry*. Berlin: Springer.
Thompson, R. A. (1974) *The Practice of Clinical Immunology*. London: Arnold.
Thompson, R. A. (Ed.) (1977) *Techniques in Clinical Immunology*. Oxford: Blackwell.
Weir, D. M. (1977) *Handbook of Experimental Immunology*. 3rd Edition. Oxford: Blackwell.
Wilkinson, A. E. (1970) The positive Wassermann reaction; investigation and interpretation. *Br. J. hosp. Med.*, **4,** 47.
Williams, C. A. & Chase, M. W. (1968) *Methods in Immunology and Immunochemistry*. New York: Academic Press.
Wright, R. W. (1970) The Australia (hepatitis) antigen. *Br. J. hosp. Med.*, **4,** 75.

Index

(Page numbers in **bold** indicate the location of the main discussion of a subject.)